Sheila Buff tells you how to eat your favorite foods and stay under your maximum daily calorie intake. Using her fantastic calorie-cutting tips, food substitutions, and calorie-burning exercises, along with her complete calorie counter, you can lose weight steadily, every day, and then keep it off forever.

DO YOU KNOW . . .

Which has fewer calories: a bottle of Bud or a glass of white wine?

Beer contains 147 calories for 12 fl. oz. White wine has 70 calories for 3.5 fl. oz. You will probably drink less wine, but ounce for ounce it has more calories (238 calories for 12 fl. oz.). Go ahead and have your beer (147 calories for 12 fl. oz.)!

Where's your chalupa when it comes to calories?

It's going to be on your hips! One chalupa averages about 400 calories. If you have a Mexican food craving, switch to tacos, which average around 200 calories and cut your intake in half!

Should you get pepperoni on that pizza?

It adds about 50 calories per slice. You be the judge.

Baking a potato? Which has more calories, white or sweet?

Surprise! A white potato baked with the skin, no toppings, equals 220 calories. A baked sweet potato is just 117 calories. But watch out what you add! Butter is 36 calories per pat, and worse, a baked potato with broccoli and cheese is 470!

The
ULTIMATE
CALORIE
COUNTER

SHEILA BUFF

St. Martin's Paperbacks

THE ULTIMATE CALORIE COUNTER

Copyright © 2002 by Sheila Buff.

All rights reserved. No part of this book may be used or reproduced in any manner whatsoever without written permission except in the case of brief quotations embodied in critical articles or reviews. For information address St. Martin's Press, 175 Fifth Avenue, New York, NY 10010.

ISBN: 0-312-98182-1

Printed in the United States of America

St. Martin's Paperbacks edition / September 2002

St. Martin's Paperbacks are published by St. Martin's Press, 175 Fifth Avenue, New York, NY 10010.

10 9 8 7 6 5 4 3

CONTENTS

The
ULTIMATE
CALORIE
COUNTER

Chapter One

CALORIES COUNT

Are you overweight? You're not alone. Today more than half of all adult Americans weigh at least 20 percent more than their ideal weight, and nearly a quarter of them weigh far more than that.

Would you like to lose weight? You're not alone there either. At any given time, about a quarter of all adult Americans are on a diet. Americans spend $33 *billion* annually on weight-loss products and services, but despite all that money, the number of overweight people continues to rise.

In today's world of fast-food restaurants, convenience foods, and busy schedules that leave little time for exercise, it's all too easy to become overweight by taking in too many calories and using too few. Reversing the process isn't quite as easy, but it's nowhere near as hard as you might think. In fact, you don't even have to go on a diet to do it. All you have to do is reduce your daily calorie intake by a small amount and increase your daily activity, also by just a small amount each day. When you take in fewer calories than you use—even by a small amount— you lose weight, steadily, safely, and for good.

What you're doing is counting calories, a weight-loss approach that is the simplest and probably most successful method of all. Teaching you how to track your daily calories and cut back on them easily is what this book is all about.

WHAT'S A CALORIE?

If you're going to lose weight the calorie-counting way, a good place to start is by understanding exactly what a calorie is.

A calorie is a unit of energy. To be precise, 1 calorie is the amount of heat (another way of saying energy) it takes to raise the temperature of 1 gram of water by 1 degree Celsius. So, if you burned a chocolate chip cookie completely and measured the amount of heat it gave off, you could then figure out how many calories the cookie contained. As it turns out, the cookie will give off about 50,000 calories. When dealing with the calories in foods, though, nutritionists make the numbers easier to deal with by giving them in kilocalories. There are 1,000 calories in 1 kilocalorie, so our chocolate chip cookie contains 50 kilocalories (abbreviated Kcal). The kilo part of kilocalories gets dropped when it comes to food labels and the like, so for all practical purposes our chocolate chip cookie is said to contain 50 calories.

By measuring the number of calories in a food, we're actually measuring how much energy that food contains. The foods we eat are made up of three basic components: carbohydrates (starches and sugars), protein, and fat. **There are 4 calories in every gram of carbohydrate and protein, and there are 9 calories in every gram of fat.** So, the 50 calories in that chocolate chip cookie come from the sugar and flour (carbohydrates), the eggs and milk (protein), and the vegetable oil (fat) that are in it.

Your body converts the food you eat into energy to keep you alive and moving. More calories mean more energy—but only up to a point. Take in as many calories as you expend, and your body weight will stay the same. Take in more calories than you expend, however, and you will gain weight as your body stores the extra energy as fat. But if you take in fewer calories than you expend, you will lose weight as your body burns fat to make up for the missing energy.

To gain 1 extra pound of weight, you have to take in approximately 3,500 more calories than you expend. And to lose 1 pound of weight, you have to expend approximately 3,500 more calories than you take in.

Don't panic—3,500 calories may sound like an impossibly big number, but it really isn't. To lose a pound in a week, you'll need to expend 500 more calories every day than you take in. That actually gives you a lot of flexibility. You could cut 500 calories from your daily diet, but that probably would mean feeling hungry all week. It's much simpler to cut just 250 calories from your daily intake and increase your activity level by another 250 calories.

As you'll discover from the calorie counter in Chapter 6, it's easy to cut 250 calories from your diet. There are about 250 calories in just two ounces of potato chips, in just one candy bar, or in just three Oreos. As you'll learn in Chapter 3, there are plenty of delicious, low-calorie substitutes for junk-food snacks. And by replacing empty calories in your diet with high-quality ones, you'll be getting better overall nutrition while you lose weight.

It's also easy to increase your activity level by 250 calories. As you'll learn in Chapter 4 on exercise, a 30-minute walk not only burns off about 130 calories, it gives you a lot of other health benefits as well. Sneak in some additional exercise besides your walk—take the stairs instead of the elevator, for example—and you're well on your way to using more calories than you take in. The result is weight loss. It's that simple.

HOW MANY CALORIES DO YOU NEED?

Before you decide how many daily calories you should eliminate from your diet, figure out how many you need to take in. About 66 percent of the calories you eat each day go to keep your body functioning normally. These are the calories that you use to keep your heart beating, your lungs breathing, your digestive system working, and so on. You burn them even when you're sleeping. About 10 percent of the calories you take in go for digesting and metabolizing your food. The rest go toward physical activity—all the moving around you do as a normal part of your daily activities. Most of your leftover calories are stored in your body as fat.

How many calories do you need each day to maintain your current weight? That depends a lot on who you are and how active you are, but you can use a simple formula to get a pretty good idea.

Let's start with what nutritionists call your basal metabolism rate (BMR). That's the number of calories you need just to maintain your basic body functions and stay alive. To find your BMR if you're a woman, take your current weight in pounds and multiply it by 10. If you're a man, multiply your current weight by 11. The result is your basal metabolism rate. So, a woman who weighs 145 pounds has a BMR of 1,450 calories a day (145 × 10 = 1,450). A man who weighs 180 pounds has a BMR of 1,980 calories a day (180 × 11 = 1,980).

To figure out how many calories you need each day beyond your BMR, you'll need to estimate how active you are, using a measure called the lifestyle percentage (L%). This number is found by estimating how active you are as a percentage of your basal metabolism rate. It's less complicated than it sounds. Start by finding the lifestyle percentage that best fits your activity level:

- **Sedentary** (lifestyle with little physical activity): Your L% is 20 percent of your BMR.

- **Somewhat active:** Your L% is 30 percent of your BMR.

- **Moderately active:** Your L% is 40 percent of your BMR.

- **Very active:** Your L% is 50 percent of your BMR.

To determine your daily calorie needs, add your BMR and your lifestyle percentage together.

So, going back to our example, let's assume you're a somewhat active 145-pound woman. Your BMR is 1,450 calories a day, and your lifestyle percentage is 30 percent of that, or an additional 435 calories (1,450 × .30 = 435). Add your BMR and your lifestyle percentage together, and you come up with a daily calorie total of 1,885 (1,450 + 435 = 1,885). That's the number of calories you need each day to maintain yourself at your current level of weight and activity.

As a rough rule of thumb, you can estimate that a moderately active woman needs about 2,000 calories a day and a moderately active man needs about 2,500 calories a day. Eat more calories than that or become less active, and you'll gain weight. Eat more *and* become less active, and you'll gain weight faster. The opposite is also true. Eat fewer calories or become more active, and you'll lose weight. Eat less *and* become more active, and you'll lose weight faster.

The combination of reduced calorie intake and increased activity is the true secret of painless, permanent weight loss. When you learn how to count your daily calories and keep them to the right number for you, you'll be able to balance your energy equation and control your weight.

ARE YOU OVERWEIGHT?

Before you start counting calories to lose weight, it's important to have an accurate idea of exactly how overweight you are. That will help you set a realistic goal for weight loss and help you maintain your new weight.

Traditionally, the ideal weight for your height was determined by a table originally compiled by the Metropolitan Life Insurance Company. The table gave weights depending on your frame—light, medium, or heavy. That's a pretty subjective measurement, however, because you can't

Table 1.1 Weight-for-Height Chart		
Height	Weight in Pounds	
	19 to 34 years	Over 35 years
5 ft 0 in	97–128	108–138
5 ft 1 in	101–132	111–143
5 ft 2 in	104–137	115–148
5 ft 3 in	107–141	119–152
5 ft 4 in	111–146	122–157
5 ft 5 in	114–150	126–162
5 ft 6 in	118–155	130–167
5 ft 7 in	121–160	134–172
5 ft 8 in	125–164	138–178
5 ft 9 in	129–169	142–183
5 ft 10 in	132–174	146–188
5 ft 11 in	136–179	151–194
6 ft 0 in	140–184	155–199
6 ft 1 in	144–189	159–205
6 ft 2 in	148–195	164–210
6 ft 3 in	152–200	168–216
6 ft 4 in	156–205	173–222
6 ft 5 in	160–211	177–228
6 ft 6 in	164–216	182–234

Source: U.S. Department of Agriculture

really know if you have "heavy" bones. Also, the Metropolitan Life table didn't take your age into account. A
somewhat better table based on your height, weight, and
age comes from the U.S. Department of Agriculture. As
shown in Table 1.1, it's a useful tool for giving you a rough
idea of what your weight should be.

The weight-for-height chart takes a one-size-fits-all approach that's not very realistic—the range within the normal weight for your height is around 30 pounds. Because
the range is so large, the chart doesn't really help you figure
out if you're normal weight, overweight, or obese.

A more accurate way to figure out if you're overweight
is to measure the amount of body fat you have. Men with

Table 1.2 Body Mass Index (BMI) Table

Height (inches)	Body Weight (pounds) 19	20	21	22	23	24	25	26	27	28	29	30	35	40
58	91	96	100	105	110	115	119	124	129	134	138	143	167	191
59	94	99	104	109	114	119	124	128	133	138	143	148	173	198
60	97	102	107	112	118	123	128	133	138	143	148	153	179	204
61	100	106	111	116	122	127	132	137	143	148	153	158	185	211
62	104	109	115	120	126	131	136	142	147	153	158	164	191	218
63	107	113	118	124	130	135	141	146	152	158	163	169	197	225
64	110	116	122	128	134	140	145	151	157	163	169	174	204	232
65	114	120	126	132	138	144	150	156	162	168	174	180	210	240
66	118	124	130	136	142	148	155	151	167	173	179	186	216	247
67	121	127	134	140	146	153	159	166	172	178	185	191	223	255
68	125	131	138	144	151	158	164	171	177	184	190	197	230	262
69	128	135	142	149	155	162	169	176	182	189	196	203	236	270
70	132	139	146	153	160	167	174	181	188	195	202	207	243	278
71	136	143	150	157	165	172	179	186	193	200	208	215	250	286
72	140	147	154	162	169	177	184	191	199	206	213	221	258	294
73	144	151	159	166	174	182	189	197	204	212	219	227	265	302
74	148	155	163	171	179	186	194	202	210	218	225	233	272	311
75	152	160	168	176	184	192	200	208	216	224	232	240	279	319
76	156	164	172	180	189	197	205	213	221	230	238	246	287	328

[Handwritten annotations: "overweight" spanning columns 26–29, "obese" near 30, "sev obese" near 40; "5 Ft" at left near rows 59–60; circles around heights 63 and 64.]

Source: National Institutes of Health

more than 25 percent body fat are obese; women with more than 30 percent body fat are obese. Measuring your body fat is a little tricky, however. It takes some special equipment and even then it's not always accurate.

Ever since 1998, doctors have used the simple body weight guidelines issued by the National Institutes of Health. These guidelines are based on your body mass index (BMI). The BMI compares your height to your weight to help figure out the amount of fat you have compared to the amount of muscle, bone, and other tissue in your body. It's a more realistic assessment, because it measures the proportion of your body that is fat and helps you determine exactly how overweight you are.

You can use a fairly complex formula to figure out your BMI, but it's a lot simpler to just look it up in Table 1.2.

Find your height in inches in the left-hand column, then look across to find your weight. Use the BMI numbers at the top of the chart to find your body mass index. If your BMI is between 20 and 24.9, you're at a normal weight for your height. If your BMI is between 25 and 29.9, you're overweight. A BMI of 30 and up means you're obese, and if your BMI is over 40, you are severely obese. (The term "morbidly obese" is sometimes used for people who are so overweight that their weight interferes with basic physical functions such as breathing.)

Using the chart, a woman who is 64 inches tall (5 feet 4 inches) and weighs anywhere between 110 and 145 pounds is within the normal weight range for her height. Ideally, though, she'd want her BMI to be in the 20 to 22 range, or between 116 and 128 pounds. The advantage of the BMI chart is that you can easily see how close you are to being overweight and get a better picture of what a healthier weight range would be for you.

There are some limitations to the BMI chart. If you're very muscular, your BMI may fall into the overweight category, even though you're very fit and healthy. Elderly people who have lost muscle mass and body fat from illness may fall into the healthy category, even though they're actually quite frail and should weigh more. For the average person under age 70, however, the BMI is a good indication of where your weight is compared to the normal range.

YOUR WAIST MEASUREMENT

If you're a woman with a waist measurement of more than 35 inches or a man with a waist measurement of more than 40, you're more likely to develop heart disease, high blood pressure, diabetes, and certain types of cancers. You can get a more accurate idea of how much more at risk you are from another important measurement of your weight: your waist-to-hip ratio (WHR). Research has shown that "apples"—people who carry their extra weight around their middles—are more likely to develop health problems associated with overweight. "Pears"—people who carry their extra weight around their thighs and buttocks—are less likely to have health problems from being overweight, although they are more likely to develop arthritis and back problems. Fortunately, apples generally find it easier than pears to lose their extra pounds. Men tend to be apples and women tend to be pears, but that's not a hard-and-fast rule. Women who gain weight after menopause tend to be apple shape.

To figure out your WHR, use a tape measure to find your waist measurement. (Measure around your torso just above your belly button.) Then find your hip measurement. (Measure around the widest part of your rear end.) Divide your waist measurement (the smaller number) by your hip measurement (the larger number). The result is your WHR. If your WHR is less than 1, you're a pear. If your WHR is 1 or more, you're an apple. A woman with a 35-inch waist and 46-inch hips is a pear, because she has a WHR of 0.76 ($35 \div 46 = 0.76$). While pears tend to have fewer of the health problems associated with being overweight, carrying too much weight around is bad for your health no matter where it is.

OVERWEIGHT AND YOUR HEALTH

People who are overweight or obese put their health at very serious risk. If you're 40 percent overweight (your BMI is over 30), you're twice as likely to die prematurely as someone the same age who's normal weight. You're also much more likely to develop life-threatening medical conditions, including diabetes, heart disease, high blood pressure, and stroke. In fact, 90 percent of the people who have adult-onset diabetes (also called Type 2 or non–insulin-dependent diabetes) are overweight. Complications from diabetes, including heart disease, kidney disease, and stroke, are the sixth leading cause of death in the United States.

Obesity is also associated with higher rates of certain

types of cancer. Obese men are more likely than normal-weight men to die from cancer of the colon, rectum, and prostate. Obese women are more likely than normal-weight women to die from cancer of the breast, uterus, cervix, and ovaries.

Some of the other health problems linked to obesity include gallbladder disease and gallstones, osteoarthritis (joint deterioration), and gout. In addition, if you're obese you may develop sleep apnea, or interrupted breathing during sleep. Sleep apnea causes loud snoring and daytime sleepiness and can lead to heart rhythm problems and high blood pressure.

LOSE A LITTLE, GAIN A LOT

The good news about your health is that losing even a small amount of weight—as little as 10 pounds—can lead to a noticeable improvement in how you feel and in your long-term health. If you have high cholesterol, for example, losing 10 pounds could lower your total cholesterol by about 16 percent—an amount that could bring your high cholesterol number back down into the normal range. If you have high blood pressure, every 2 pounds you lose translates into a 2-point drop in both your systolic and diastolic blood pressure. Losing 10 pounds means your blood pressure might drop about 10 points. That might not put you back in the normal range, but it could mean a reduction in the amount of medication you need to take. In many cases, overweight people with high blood pressure can stop taking medicine for it if they lower their weight by 10 percent. If you weigh 200 pounds, that means losing 20 pounds.

Overweight people are twice as likely to develop adult-onset diabetes as people who are normal weight. The heavier you are, the greater your risk—even being at the high end of the normal weight range nearly triples your diabetes risk compared to people at the low end.

Studies have shown that nine out of 10 cases of adult-onset diabetes could be prevented by losing weight and exercising more. If you already have diabetes, losing as little as 5 to 10 percent of your body weight could do a lot to help control your blood sugar level, reduce your need for medication, and lower the chances of long-term diabetes problems such as heart disease, kidney disease, amputation, and blindness.

IT'S IN MY GENES

Obesity tends to run in families, but is that because you share "fat genes" or because you share eating and lifestyle habits? It's probably some of both. Your genes do play a role in your weight, and if there are many overweight people in your family, you'll be more likely to be overweight as well. If members of your family have developed health problems related to being overweight, such as diabetes, you're more likely to develop them too if you're overweight or even on the heavy end of the normal weight range.

You're not genetically doomed to a life of fatness, however. Your environment plays a big part as well. You can't change your genes, but you certainly can be aware of them and change what you eat and how active you are.

WHAT IS SAFE WEIGHT LOSS?

Slow and steady weight loss of 1 to 2 pounds a week is the safest and surest way to lose weight. Why? Because the only way to lose a pound or two a week is to make simple, long-term changes in your eating habits and activity level. No crash diets, no weird food restrictions, no rapid weight loss followed by equally rapid weight gain—just small, positive changes you can live with on a permanent basis.

ASK YOUR DOCTOR

Before you start on a weight-loss program or start to become more physically active, visit your doctor for a checkup. You need to be sure that your weight gain isn't caused by a health problem such as an underactive thyroid gland (hypothyroidism) or depression. Some drugs, including birth control pills, hormone replacement therapy to treat menopause symptoms, steroids, and some antidepressants can be an underlying cause of weight gain. You also need to be sure that increasing your level of physical activity will be safe for you, and you need to know if there are any restrictions on the types of activities you can do.

As part of your examination your doctor will take your blood pressure, check your heart, and measure your blood cholesterol levels and the amount of glucose in your blood (a marker for diabetes). The results will be your baseline numbers—the numbers that losing weight will almost certainly improve.

At the end of your checkup your doctor may ask you to come back in three to six months. If you lose 1 pound a week for six months, you will lose 21 pounds between this visit and your next. When those baseline numbers are checked again, there is a very good chance that they will be sharply improved. There's no better proof of how weight loss helps your health.

PREVENTING GALLSTONES

Although weight loss will improve your health in almost every way, there is one health problem that is of real concern if you lose weight improperly. Gallstones are a painful and serious health problem that can affect dieters, especially if they lose weight rapidly.

Gallstones are clumps of solid material that accumulate in your gallbladder, a small, pear-shape organ in your abdomen. Your gallbladder contains bile, a fluid made by your liver and used in digestion. As food passes from your stomach to your small intestine, your gallbladder contracts and releases bile through ducts into the intestine. If a gallstone gets stuck in the bile duct, the result is severe pain and possibly surgery to remove the gallbladder. Every year in the United States there are more than 600,000 hospitalizations for gallstones and over 500,000 operations to remove gallbladders.

Being overweight is a strong risk factor for gallstones. In fact, a woman with a BMI of 30 or more has at least double the risk of developing gallstones as a woman with a BMI of 25 or less.

For reasons researchers still don't understand, however, losing weight actually increases your odds of having a gallstone. If you lose weight rapidly or follow a very-low-calorie diet, your odds go up even more. Gradual weight loss, the kind you get by counting calories, may help reduce your risk of getting gallstones.

The risk of gallstones from rapid weight loss is real, but it's still small—about 4 to 6 percent. The risk if you lose weight gradually is probably even less. And while you do have a small chance of getting gallstones from weight loss, you have an almost certain chance of getting diabetes, heart disease, high blood pressure, and other potentially fatal health problems if you stay overweight.

WEIGHING YOURSELF

You may have noticed that your weight seems to vary a bit depending on what time of day you weigh yourself and also on which scale you use. Your weight at your doctor's office, standing on an expensive beam scale, is probably different from the weight you get on your bathroom scale.

As long as you weigh yourself on the same scale at the same time of day, it doesn't matter which weight is your "true" weight. What matters is that each time you step on that scale, you weigh a little bit less than you did the time before.

If you weigh yourself every day, you won't really be able to detect your weight loss if you're losing a pound a week. Most scales can't detect a difference of just a few ounces from day to day. Weight-loss specialists recommend that you weigh yourself only once a week or even less often. Do it first thing in the morning, without any clothes on, and always use the same scale. Keep a written record of the date and your weight. For extra encouragement, keep a running total of all the weight you've lost.

ALL ABOUT YOU

Before you begin counting calories, write down some basic information about yourself, as shown on the sample data sheet on pages 16–17. Write down your height and weight, and then use the Body Mass Index table to find your current BMI. Figure out your waist-to-hip ratio as well. Write down the baseline information you've gotten from your doctor about your cholesterol levels, your blood sugar, and your blood pressure. Next, put your personal data sheet away someplace safe and don't look at it for a month.

After you've been counting calories for a month, weigh yourself, figure out your BMI and WHR, and write it all down on your data sheet. Compare your new data to your old and see if there's been any improvement. You've probably lost a few pounds by now, and you might even have moved into a lower BMI number.

As you continue to count calories and lose weight, record your personal data once a month on the data sheet. In a few months' time you should see an encouraging trend of continuing weight loss. When you go back to your doctor after six months or so, you may see that your new cholesterol and blood pressure numbers are also moving into a healthier range. If you've been diagnosed with high blood sugar or diabetes, those numbers may be improved as well.

Let's face it—weight loss is a slow process. It can get discouraging sometimes, but if you keep records, you can see that you're making progress, even if it's only a few pounds a month.

PRESCRIPTION WEIGHT LOSS

Wouldn't it be great if you could take a magic pill and lose weight? That's what a lot of people thought when Pondimin® (fenfluramine hydrochloride) and Redux® (dexfenfluramine hydrochloride) were introduced in 1995. Hailed as the miracle solution to obesity, these drugs were taken off the market in 1997 after they were shown to cause serious heart problems in some patients. Today the only prescription drug designed specifically for weight loss is Xenical® (orlistat). This drug works in your intestines by blocking about a third of your absorption of dietary fat. There are some serious drawbacks to Xenical®, though, including digestive problems. It's not a long-term solution for permanent weight loss, but when it's combined with a low-calorie diet, it can help start you down the weight-loss path and keep you on it. Some people find that antidepressants such as Prozac© (fluoxetine) help them control their appetites and stick to a healthier eating plan. If you think medication might help you, discuss your weight-loss plans with your doctor.

DIET PILLS AND DIET SCAMS

The shelves of any health-food store are crammed with all sorts of pills, teas, and supplements that claim to help you lose weight. The labels say that whatever is inside will burn fat faster, or block fat, or melt fat away. Will it? Of course not.

Be very cautious about these so-called shortcuts to weight loss. They won't really help you lose weight, and

Personal Data Sheet

NAME:		AGE:		HEIGHT:
Date	Weight	BMI	Waist/Hip Ratio	Blood Pressure

Total Cholesterol	LDL Cholesterol	HDL Cholesterol	Triglycerides	Blood Sugar	Other

they could be dangerous to your health. Just read the warnings and possible side effects of over-the-counter diet pills, such as Acutrim®, and you'll understand why these drugs should be avoided. Herbal weight-loss supplements and teas often contain ephedra (also called ma huang), a stimulant that has been linked to a number of deaths. Other diet teas contain diuretic herbs such as uva ursi (also called buchu or bearberry) that increase urination. The water loss makes you lose a few pounds quickly, but at the price of possible dehydration and kidney damage. Remember, just because a product is "natural" or "herbal" doesn't mean it's safe or that it works.

Nonprescription fat-blockers such as chitosan are said to work by binding fat in your intestines, but as with prescription Xenical®, there are some serious drawbacks to this approach to weight loss. Chitosan can cause intestinal discomfort, including gas, cramping, and leakage. And as with Xenical®, just taking the supplement won't cause long-term weight loss unless you also change your eating patterns.

Because so many people are eager to lose weight, they are easy targets for scam artists peddling fad diets and "miracle weight-loss systems." Watch out for anything related to weight loss if it promises you a quick fix, bans whole categories of foods, or is based on selling you some sort of product or supplement. If you fall for one of these scams, the only thing that will lose weight will be your wallet.

VERY-LOW-CALORIE DIETS

If you're very overweight and you need to have significant short-term weight loss, your doctor may prescribe a very-low-calorie diet (VLCD). When you're on a VLCD, you drink a commercially prepared formula containing less than 800 calories a day instead of eating your usual meals. These formulas aren't the same as over-the-counter meal replacements, such as Slim•Fast®, which are meant to be substituted for one or two meals a day. (See Chapter 5 for more on Slim•Fast®.)

VLCDs are definitely not the way to permanent weight loss. You'd go on such an extreme diet only if your BMI is over 30 and if your doctor prescribes it. Very-low-calorie diets are used only to treat medical complications of obesity, such as breathing difficulties or if your excess body fat would complicate needed surgery.

GETTING STARTED

If you're ready to get started on the path to permanent weight loss, you're ready to start counting calories. But before you do, make sure this is a good time for you. Is the food-rich holiday season coming up? Are you scheduled for a lot of business travel or a vacation? Is anything highly stressful coming up in your life? Are you pregnant or having a serious health problem? It's hard to stick to counting calories under these circumstances, especially if you're new to this approach. Don't sabotage yourself. Pick a relatively calm and healthy time in your life to start calorie counting.

Ask yourself one final question: Why do I want to lose weight? The desire to lose weight has to come from inside you. If you're dieting because you're getting pressure from family members, friends, or your doctor, the chances are good that you won't keep the weight off. It's only when you lose weight for yourself, not others, that dieting works in the long run.

Are you ready? It's time to learn the easy, practical way to count calories for weight loss.

Chapter Two

CALORIE COUNTING THE SANE AND SIMPLE WAY

Counting your daily calories is a simple and nutritionally balanced approach to weight loss. Once you get the hang of it, you'll see how easy it is to track your daily intake of calories. You'll soon be able to see where the extra calories are coming from, and you'll learn how to replace them without ever going hungry.

WHY CALORIE COUNTING WORKS

Calorie counting works for a lot of reasons, but the main one is that you can eat anything you want. You're not restricted to a small number of foods, and whole categories of foods aren't off limits. Because there are so many delicious, satisfying low-calorie foods, you never have to go hungry. When you count calories, you get good nutrition—unlike fad diets, which are almost always unbalanced and unhealthful. Because you can choose from so many foods, you never get so bored by your diet that you have cravings for forbidden foods or stop dieting altogether. In fact, once you've become an experienced calorie counter and start losing that excess weight, you can even cheat on your diet now and then.

Calorie counting is inexpensive—no special prepared foods, drink mixes, or diet bars; no supplements or drugs; no organization to join. Best of all, you can count calories on your own, without trying to fit dieting meetings into your busy schedule.

CALORIE-COUNTING BASICS

Eat more calories than you use, and you'll gain weight. Use more calories than you eat, and you'll lose weight.

That's the general idea. Now let's get down to specifics.

• If you take in 3,500 more calories than you use, you will gain 1 pound of fat. Use 3,500 more calories than you eat, and you'll lose 1 pound of fat.

• Keep your calorie intake below 2,000 calories a day if you're a woman and below 2,500 calories a day if you're a man, and you'll lose weight.

• Reduce your calorie intake to 1,600 calories a day if you're a woman and 2,000 calories a day if you're a man, and you will lose weight steadily and safely without hunger pangs.

• Cut your daily intake by just 250 calories a day and you will lose 25 pounds in a year.

When you first start counting your calories, you may be amazed to realize how many calories you eat each day. But when you look at the calorie counts for common foods in Chapter 6, it's all too easy to see how 3,500 extra calories can creep into your diet over the course of just a few days.

Let's look at the calorie counts of a typical day in the life of a typical woman who weighs 30 pounds too much:

• **Breakfast:** Coffee with sugar and milk (40 calories), a bowl of cornflakes with milk (175 calories), a glass of orange juice (90 calories), and a banana (105 calories). Total calories: 410.

- **Coffee break:** Coffee with sugar and milk (40 calories) and a jelly doughnut (220 calories). Total calories: 260. Total calories for the day so far: 670.

- **Lunch:** Cheeseburger (310 calories), large fries (400 calories), and a milkshake (320 calories) at a fast-food restaurant. Add it all up and she's taken in 1,030 calories—and that's just lunch. Total calories for the day so far: 1,700.

- **Afternoon snack:** 5 chocolate chip cookies (250 calories). Total calories for the day so far: 1,950, or the maximum an average woman can eat without gaining weight.

- **Dinner:** 2 slices pepperoni pizza (440 calories), salad with ranch dressing (50 calories), 2 dinner rolls with butter (240 calories), 1 can of cola (100 calories), and a big scoop of butter pecan ice cream (460). Calories for the meal: 1,150. Total calories for the day so far: 3,330.

- **Evening snack:** 6 ounces of potato chips (900 calories), another can of cola (100 calories). Total calories: 1,000.

The grand total of a day's worth of calories: 4,330, or 2,330 more calories than a typical woman needs. And 2,330 calories translate into more than half a pound of weight gain. Average that out for a week and our typical woman has gained 3.5 pounds. Even if she cuts back by 500 calories a day, she'll still gain weight, at the rate of a bit more than 2 pounds a week.

It doesn't have to be this way. Our imaginary woman could easily have eaten under 2,000 calories for the day without ever feeling hungry—and gotten better nutrition to boot. Here's how:

- **Breakfast:** Coffee with artificial sweetener and nonfat milk (10 calories), a bowl of cornflakes with nonfat milk (140 calories), a glass of orange juice (90 calories), and an apple (80 calories). Total calories: 320. Calories saved: 90.

• **Coffee break:** Coffee with artificial sweetener and nonfat milk (10 calories), another apple (80 calories), and 2 chocolate crunch rice cakes (100 calories). Total calories: 190. Calories saved: 70. Total calories for the day so far: 510. Total calories saved so far: 160.

• **Lunch:** Cheeseburger (310 calories), small fries (220 calories), and a diet soda (10 calories) at a fast-food restaurant. Total calories: 540. Calories saved: 490. Total calories for the day so far: 1,000. Total calories saved so far: 700.

• **Afternoon snack:** 3 chocolate crunch rice cakes (150 calories). Total calories for the day so far: 1,150. Total calories saved so far: 800.

• **Dinner:** 2 slices pepperoni pizza (440 calories), salad with nonfat ranch dressing (35 calories), 1 cup steamed broccoli (50 calories), 1 dinner roll with butter (140 calories), and 1 can of diet cola (no calories). Calories for the meal: 665. Total calories saved: 165. Total calories for the day so far: 1,675.

• **Evening snack:** Large bowl of sugar-free strawberry-flavored gelatin (40 calories), another can of diet cola (no calories). Total calories: 40. Calories saved: 960. Total calories for the day: 1,715.

A typical woman who is moderately active will lose somewhere between ½ and 1 pound a week if she eats only 1,715 calories a day.

Is there a big difference between the two menus? Yes and no. Both menus have a lot of the same foods, including cheeseburgers and fries. But by having slightly smaller portions of some foods and making some very simple substitutions—nonfat milk for whole milk, diet soda for a milkshake, an apple instead of a doughnut, gelatin for potato chips—the number of calories is cut by 1,925 calories, or more than half. And even though our typical woman is actually eating far fewer calories, her nutrition is much better, because she's eating more fresh fruit and vegetables and less high-fat junk food.

COUNTING YOUR CALORIES

How many calories are you taking in each day? Probably more than you think. Study after study has shown that people consistently underestimate their daily calorie intake.

It's not surprising that they do, because today we have a very distorted idea of what a portion is. To take a good example, a plain bagel has 195 calories—but only if it has a diameter of 3½ inches or weighs about 4 ounces, the standard size used by nutritionists. The bagel you buy from the coffee cart at break time probably is considerably larger than that, with proportionately more calories.

Even when your portions are the usual size, it's easy to forget the little things that go along with them. If you put an ounce of cream cheese on that plain bagel, you're adding 99 calories to the total, bringing it up to 294 calories.

YOUR FOOD DIARY

The one and only way you can discover your real calorie intake is to keep a food diary. Record *everything* you eat when you eat it. Don't rely on your memory at the end of the day—as the example of the bagel above shows, it's too easy to forget about the extra calories that make the difference between losing weight and staying the same or even gaining. It's also very easy to forget about all those between-meal snacks.

Try to be as honest and accurate as you can when you write down what you eat. If you leave things out, you won't get a fair idea of what you're really eating, and you won't lose weight.

Calculate the calories using the calorie counter in Chapter 6. You don't have to be accurate to the last calorie. Rounding out the numbers is OK—all you need to do is get a good approximate idea of how many calories you consume each day. After you've been keeping your diary for a week or so, you'll have a pretty fair idea of what your average daily calorie intake really is.

Looking up the calorie counts is quick and easy. Once you get the hang of it, keeping your food diary takes only a few minutes a day. You can speed things up by keeping a short list of the calorie counts for the foods you eat most often. For example, most people tend to eat the same things for breakfast, so once you've figured out the calories in your usual breakfast, that number will tend to stay about the same from day to day.

After counting your calories for only a few days, you'll probably be amazed to see what your true intake is. You may well realize, for instance, that your between-meal eating adds up to as many calories as your main meals. Keeping a daily food diary helps you discover where all those extra calories are coming from. Once you know that, you can easily make simple diet changes that will cut your calories but leave you feeling well fed and satisfied. (See Chapter 3 for practical tips on cutting calories without cutting taste or nutrition.)

The sample diary sheets on pages 37–39 are a good way to track your daily calories. They have plenty of space to record your meals and snacks. Make lots of copies, because you'll need to keep your food diary on an ongoing basis over the next year or so.

Write down *everything* you eat *when* you eat it—no exceptions. (If you wait until later, you'll probably forget to include some items, especially snacks.) Give the amount or portion size whenever possible (3 cookies, 1 orange, 2 breadsticks, and so on).

You don't have to carry your diary sheets around with you. You may find it easier to record your food intake in a small notebook or on an index card that fits easily into your pocket or purse. Then you can fill out your food diary form and estimate your calories at the end of the day.

The sample diary has eight check-off boxes for your water intake. In Chapter 3 you'll learn why it's so important to drink at least eight glasses of water or other liquid each day. The check-off boxes make it easier for you to keep yourself on track.

The sample diary also has space for you to record your exercise level for the day. As you'll learn in Chapter 4, cutting calories is only half the solution—increasing your activity level is the essential other half.

Keeping a food diary helps you grasp an important advantage of the calorie-counting approach to weight loss. To lose weight, you need to cut your daily intake by an *average* of about 250 calories a day. That means that when you have one of those days where you just have to have a candy bar, you can make up for it the next day by being a little more careful. You can also help balance out a high-calorie day by exercising more that day or the next. Use your food diary to keep track of your calorie intake and your exercise level. As long as your food diary shows that over a week you are averaging 250 calories fewer a day, each individual day isn't that important.

COUNT CALORIES OR COUNT FAT?

One gram of protein or carbohydrate has 4 calories, while 1 gram of fat has 9 calories. You might think, then, that cutting back on calories from fat would be the best way to lose weight. In fact, cutting fat and not really thinking about your overall calorie intake is the basis for some popular diet plans, such as the T-Factor diet.

Cutting back on some fat in your diet is a good way to reduce your overall calorie intake. One 8-ounce glass of whole milk, for example, has 150 calories and 8 grams of fat. An equal amount of skim milk has just 86 calories and less than ½ gram of fat. That's a savings of 64 calories, and you're still getting the important calcium and vitamins from the milk. One cup of low-fat strawberry yogurt has 240 calories and 3 grams of fat; 1 cup of no-fat strawberry yogurt has only 160 calories—a savings of 80 calories. Switching to reduced-fat or no-fat salad dressings is a good way to save some calories, and plenty of other tasty nonfat, low-fat, and reduced-fat foods are available.

The best way to cut back on your fat calories and improve your health is to avoid partially hydrogenated vegetable oil, a type of processed fat also known as trans fat or trans fatty acids. This is the worst kind of fat—gram for gram, it clogs your arteries twice as much as saturated fat. Trans fats are found in baked goods such as cookies and cakes, in french fries and other deep-fried foods, and in snack foods such as potato chips. By avoiding these high-calorie, low-nutrition foods, you're also avoiding the dangerous trans fat and saving your calories for foods that provide real nutrition.

Beware the low-fat trap, however! Just because a food has less fat doesn't always mean it has fewer calories. If you look at the calorie counts on the food labels, you'll see that low-fat cookies, for instance, often have almost as many calories as the regular version. Low-fat peanut butter has exactly the same number of calories as regular peanut butter!

The low-fat or no-fat label might fool you into eating a lot more calories than you realize. That's because the manufacturers end up adding more sugar to make up for the missing flavor from the fat. No fat doesn't mean no calories, and reduced fat doesn't always mean reduced calories. And if the low-fat version really does have fewer calories, it's all too easy to use that to justify eating more than you should of the food.

Instead of falling for low-fat versions of high-calorie, high-fat foods, skip these foods altogether. Instead of low-fat cookies, for instance, have some fresh fruit (no fat at all) instead.

Dietary fat plays a big role in helping you feel satisfied

by your food and in keeping you from getting too hungry between meals. If you cut back on dietary fat too far, you might end up eating even more calories in an effort to feel full. Several scientific studies have shown that it is much easier to stick to a diet that allows a moderate amount of fat, especially healthful fats such as olive oil.

It's also important to remember that you need some dietary fat for good nutrition—cutting your fat intake too low might actually be harmful.

In the end, watching only your fat grams probably isn't a good strategy for permanent weight loss. Cutting back on fat as just one part of your overall calorie counting will give you more food choices and keep your diet nutritionally well balanced.

CUT CALORIES, NOT NUTRITION

One of the most positive benefits of counting calories is that you actually can improve your nutrition while losing weight. Counting calories makes you realize how much junk food has found its way into your diet and teaches you how to substitute high-quality, low-calorie foods instead. Learning how to eat a well-balanced diet will help you lose weight and, more important, keep it off.

The familiar food pyramid created by the United States Department of Agriculture (USDA), shown on page 29, is a good guide to the basics of healthy eating. By following the pyramid, you get the recommended amounts of all food components, including vitamins and minerals.

Although the food pyramid isn't designed for weight loss, it is a very good framework for calorie counting. By sticking to the basic concept of the food pyramid and going with the lower number of portions within each category, you'll cut your calories while still getting well-balanced nutrition.

Let's take a closer look at the food pyramid. At the base of it are 6 to 11 servings of grains and cereals such as bread,

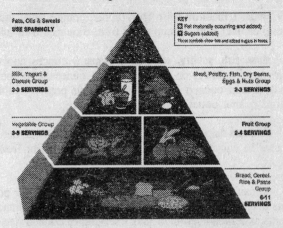

pasta, and rice. At the next level up are 3 to 5 servings of vegetables and 2 to 4 servings of fruit. Above that are 2 to 3 servings of animal foods such as meat, fish, poultry, eggs, dairy products, or of high-calorie plant foods such as beans and nuts. At the very tip of the pyramid are fats, oils, and sugars—foods that should be eaten sparingly.

Looking at the food pyramid, it might seem that you would gain weight by following it. Eleven servings of grains and cereals, for instance, is a lot to eat—or is it? Don't confuse the number of servings in the food pyramid with the size of the servings. Here's how the USDA defines a serving in each category:

• **Breads and cereals:** 1 slice bread, ½ English muffin, ½ cup cooked rice, ½ cup cooked pasta, 1 ounce breakfast cereal

• **Vegetables:** ½ cup cooked vegetables, ½ cup chopped raw vegetables, 1 cup leafy greens, 1 small potato, 6 ounces vegetable juice

• **Fruits:** 1 medium fresh fruit (apple, orange, pear, etc.), ½ cup canned fruit, ¼ cup dried fruit, 6 ounces fruit juice

• **Meat, fish, poultry, eggs, nuts, beans:** 3 ounces cooked lean meat, poultry, or fish; 2 eggs; 7 ounces tofu (bean curd); 1 cup cooked legumes (beans and peas); 4 tablespoons peanut butter, ½ cup nuts or seeds

• **Milk and dairy products:** 1 cup milk or yogurt, 1 ounce cheese, ½ cup cottage cheese, ½ cup ice cream or frozen yogurt

As you can see, the food pyramid is based on smaller portions than you might think. An English muffin, for instance, counts as 2 bread servings, and 1 serving of cooked rice or pasta is just ½ cup.

Once you understand more about the servings, the food pyramid isn't a formula for overeating at all. In fact, you can use the food pyramid as a handy way to count calories. If you want to cut back to 1,600 calories a day, choose 6 servings from the breads and grains category, 3 from the vegetables, 2 from the fruits, and 2 to 3 from the milk and dairy category. Top it off with 5 ounces from the meat, beans, or nuts category, and you've cut calories without even counting. If 1,600 calories is too low for you or if you find yourself getting too hungry between meals, increase your calories by adding additional servings from the grains and vegetables categories—these give you the most nutrition and the least fat for the calories.

PORTION CONTROL

To count your daily calories accurately, you need to learn how to estimate your intake based on the size of the portions you eat. Fortunately, in many cases, the American food industry has already done this for you. Any packaged or prepared food carries a label that tells you exactly how many calories there are in a portion—and how many of those calories come from fat, protein, carbohydrates, and added sugar. All you have to do is read it.

There's a catch to the food label, though. The portion sizes can be very, very misleading. There are 110 calories in a portion of oatmeal raisin cookies—that's just a few more calories than there are in an apple. But the cookie portion is just two smallish cookies. Will you really eat just two? Before you know it, you're likely to have eaten six cookies, for 360 calories and very little in the way of nutrition. On the other hand, two crisp, juicy apples would give you about 200 calories along with plenty of fiber, lots of vitamin C, potassium, and other good nutrients, and no fat whatsoever. You'd feel fuller longer from eating the apples.

The package label isn't always right at hand, of course, and there are no labels on restaurant foods and foods you cook yourself. That's where the calorie counter in Chapter 6 is particularly handy. Use it to look up your favorite restaurant foods and get an idea of how many calories they contain.

WOULD YOU LIKE TO NORMAL SIZE THAT?

The portions used for calorie counts tend to be smaller than the portions most people are used to eating these days. With a little practice, though, you can easily learn to size up your portion and make an accurate estimate of the calories in it.

To get a real sense of what a good portion size is, do a little experimenting in your kitchen. Give yourself a typical portion of your favorite foods, and then use a measuring cup and an inexpensive dieter's scale (or postage scale) to measure it. Then compare your portion to the serving sizes for the food pyramid. If there's a big difference, you've put your finger on one major reason for your extra weight.

Using your scale and measuring cups, measure out the recommended portions for your favorite foods. Put the portion into a bowl or plate to get an idea of what it looks like. Pretty soon you'll be able to eyeball the right portion size and know when you're eating more.

Of course, you can't always go around measuring and weighing your food. Try comparing your portion to some common objects to get an idea of the size:

- 3½ ounces of meat, fish, or poultry are about the size of a deck of cards or a bar of soap.

- 8 ounces of meat, fish, or poultry are about the size of a thin paperback book.

- 1 medium apple or orange is about the size of a tennis ball.

- 1 cup of cut fruit or berries is about the size of a baseball.

- 1 medium potato is about the size of a computer mouse.

- 1 cup of salad greens equals about 4 whole large leaves.

- 1 ounce of sliced cheese is about the size of a 3½-inch computer diskette; 1 ounce of unsliced cheese is roughly the size of a small matchbox, a domino, or your thumb.

- 1 4-ounce bagel is about the diameter of a compact disc; so are pancakes and waffles.

- 1 slice of pizza fits into a standard business envelope.

- 2 tablespoons of peanut butter are roughly the size of a golf ball.

• 1 teaspoon of butter or margarine is about the size of the tip of your thumb.

• For metric measurements: 1 gram is about 0.035 of an ounce; there are about 28 grams in an ounce and about 15 grams in a tablespoon.

With a little practice you'll easily be able to estimate portion sizes and get a rough idea of how many calories you're taking in. This is an important step for losing weight. Simply being aware of correct portion sizes and approximate calorie counts will go a long way to helping you cut back on your intake.

LOW CALORIES, HIGH NUTRITION

When you're cutting calories to lose weight, every calorie you eat really has to count. You want to get the most satisfaction and the most nutrition out of everything you eat. The two can easily go together.

The foods we eat are made up of carbohydrates (starches and sugars), protein, and fat. For a good overall diet, about half your calories should come from carbohydrates. Whenever possible, make those carbohydrates complex ones from relatively unrefined foods: starches from baked potatoes, whole-wheat pasta, brown rice, whole-wheat bread, and so on. Keep the refined carbohydrates, such as white bread, cake, sugar, and candy to a minimum—or eliminate them altogether. Protein in your diet comes from meat, poultry, fish, eggs, beans and peas, and nuts. You almost certainly need a lot less protein than you currently eat. As a rule of thumb, you need only about half a gram of protein for each pound of your body weight. If you weigh 160 pounds, then, you would need only about 80 grams of protein—or the equivalent of two roasted chicken drumsticks and two wings.

Don't cut your protein portions back too far, though. To

maintain strong bones no matter what your weight, a woman needs to eat at least 50 grams of protein a day; a man needs to eat at least 65. If you get most of your protein from vegetable foods such as soybeans, you need even more—about 70 grams a day for a woman and about 85 for a man.

The amount of fat in your diet should be no more than 30 percent of your total calories. Saturated fat, found in animal foods, should be no more than 10 percent of your calories. Saturated fat in the diet is one of the culprits behind high blood cholesterol, which can lead to heart disease. The other culprit is partially hydrogenated vegetable oil, or trans fat. When you're watching your calories, foods high in saturated fat and trans fats are the first ones to go. By doing so, you'll not only lose weight, you'll protect your heart as well.

If you eat a 2,000-calorie diet, you should be getting no more than 65 grams of fat a day, of which no more than 20 grams should come from saturated fat. If you cut back to under 2,000 calories a day, however, don't lower your total fat intake to below 65 grams. You won't feel satisfied by your food if it doesn't contain some fat. Even worse, you won't be getting enough vitamin A and vitamin E, because you need some dietary fat to absorb them. You'll be doing your heart a big favor if your 65 grams of fat come mostly from healthy unsaturated vegetable oils, such as olive oil or canola oil.

Remember that there are 9 calories to 1 gram of fat, so 65 grams of fat works out to getting 585 calories a day from fat. Use food labels and the information in the calorie counter in Chapter 6 to figure out where your fat calories are coming from and keep them under control.

THE FIBER FACTOR

Plant foods, including fruits, vegetables, nuts, and beans, contain carbohydrates, some fat, and some protein. They also contain the calorie counter's secret ingredient: fiber.

Dietary fiber comes from the indigestible parts of plant foods. Because you can't digest fiber, it doesn't have any calories. What fiber does have is bulk—it fills you up and keeps you from getting hungry too fast.

Picture yourself eating six chocolate chip cookies in a row. All too easy, isn't it? Now picture yourself eating six carrots in a row. Almost impossible. Why? Because those sweet, crunchy, no-fat carrots are full of fiber (and lots of vitamins and minerals). You'd be full long before you got to the sixth one. Not only that, the full feeling will last for a long time—you won't be hungry again for a couple of hours.

When you count calories and substitute plenty of high-fiber fruits and vegetables for high-calorie, low-fiber foods like cake, you lose weight. Numerous medical studies have shown that you gain in health at the same time. A high-fiber diet helps lower your blood cholesterol, improves your blood sugar levels, and helps keep your blood pressure down. A high-fiber diet also helps you avoid digestive problems such as constipation.

Dietary authorities all agree that everyone, not just calorie counters, should aim for 25 to 30 grams of fiber a day. That might seem like a lot, but it's not that hard to accomplish. In fact, simply by following the food pyramid servings for fruits and vegetables and making sure your starchy foods come from whole grains whenever possible, you'll get up to 25 to 30 grams of fiber a day almost without trying.

COUNTING DOWN

Counting calories means never going on a diet. Once you've learned how to track your daily calories and have figured out how to cut the excess calories from your food, you can eat anything you want. All you really need to know is that your calorie intake, on average, can't be more than whatever amount you need to lose weight or maintain your weight. What that amount will be is up to you.

The real secret to calorie counting is learning how to swap high-calorie foods for lower-calorie ones that taste just as good or better. You'll enjoy your food, you'll never be hungry, and you'll be healthier as well. Is it hard to get all those benefits? Not at all—as you'll learn in the next chapter.

My Food Diary

Date:

BREAKFAST

Food	Portion	Calories

Breakfast calories:
Calories for the day:

MORNING SNACK

Food	Portion	Calories

Snack calories:
Calories for the day:

LUNCH

Food	Portion	Calories

Lunch calories:
Calories for the day:

AFTERNOON SNACK

Food	Portion	Calories

Snack calories:

Calories for the day:

DINNER

Food	Portion	Calories

Dinner calories:

Calories for the day:

EVENING SNACK

Food	Portion	Calories

Snack calories:

Calories for the day:

TOTAL CALORIES FOR DAY:

Liquids intake (each box is one 8-ounce glass of water, diet soda (not cola), herbal tea, or
   decaffeinated beverage)

☐   ☐   ☐   ☐   ☐   ☐   ☐   ☐
1   2   3   4   5   6   7   8

Exercise:

Type of exercise:

Distance/time:

Chapter Three

PRACTICAL STRATEGIES FOR CALORIE COUNTERS

Calorie counting is a simple approach to weight loss, but as every dieter knows, weight loss is never simple. The road to a healthier, thinner you has plenty of potholes, but most can be avoided with a little knowledge. And if you do fall into a hole, it will never be so deep that you can't find your way out.

The practical advice in this chapter comes from the experience of successful calorie counters—people who have lost weight and kept it off. They did it. You can too.

SET REALISTIC GOALS

When you decide it's time to lose that extra weight, ask yourself why. Is it because you truly want to look and feel better, both for yourself and for your family? Once you've made that important decision, it's time to set yourself some realistic goals. Do you want to look like Britney Spears? It's unlikely, no matter how much weight you lose.

There's nothing wrong about wanting to improve your appearance, of course, and losing weight is a good way to do it. But think about another good reason to lose weight: your health. You'll look better, and you'll also feel better— a lot better, even if all you lose is 10 or 15 pounds. You'll also be improving your long-term health.

Give yourself a realistic, attainable weight-loss goal.

You don't have to get back down to a size 6 or lose 50 pounds in three months. It's more important—and much easier—to focus on reducing your body mass index (BMI) by just one or two levels. (Check back to Chapter 1 to learn how to calculate your BMI and what a healthy range of weight is for your height.) Each drop in your BMI is only about 10 pounds of weight, but it's much more than that in better health and appearance. Remember, numerous scientific studies have shown that losing as little as 10 to 15 pounds can greatly improve health problems such as diabetes. And if you lose just 10 or 15 pounds, people will definitely notice that you're looking better.

Once you've gotten your BMI down a couple of levels, refocus on getting it down another notch or two. The slow and steady weight loss that comes with calorie counting means that you could drop several BMI levels in less than a year. That will probably bring you well within the normal weight range. And even if it doesn't, you're definitely a lot closer.

Another way to look at realistic weight loss is that many weight-related health problems improve markedly if you lose just 5 to 10 percent of your body weight. In other words, you don't have to get down to your ideal weight in order to notice improved health—you'll feel the benefits almost at once. If you weigh 170 pounds and are suffering from high blood pressure or diabetes, for instance, all you have to lose to improve those conditions is between 8.5 and 17 pounds (5 to 10 percent of your body weight). And if losing just that amount makes you feel better, think how much better you'll feel as your weight continues to drop!

EAT EARLY AND OFTEN

A number of scientific studies have looked at what people who have successfully lost a lot of weight have in common. Two things really stand out. First, these people always start their day with a good breakfast. Second, they eat several smaller meals spaced regularly through the day. They never skip meals, and they don't eat a small lunch and then a really big dinner.

If you skip meals or eat just a small amount, you'll almost always make up for it by snacking or overeating at your next meal. You won't lose any weight by skipping meals, but you will be hungry and grouchy.

Follow the example of the people who have lost weight and kept it off. Start your day with a big, nutritious breakfast that contains carbohydrates, fiber, and some protein. You might not be able to prepare a small meal at morning and afternoon break times, but you can easily skip the doughnuts and have a substantial snack instead. Good choices would be fruit, low-fat cheese, baked chicken legs, low-fat yogurt with fruit, rice cakes, and low-fat baked crackers. You can also try diet shakes and energy bars—a recent study has shown that these meal replacers can be very helpful for people cutting calories. They're tasty and very convenient. (Meal-replacement diet programs are discussed in detail in Chapter 5.)

EAT AND WAIT

Successful dieters know that it's a long way between your stomach and your brain. Because it takes a little while for your brain to realize that your stomach has been fed, you often continue to feel hungry even after you've eaten a meal. That's when you can eat too many calories as you reach for that second portion or decide to have dessert after all. But if you wait just 15 or 20 minutes after eating, your brain will catch up with your stomach. Your hunger will disappear and you'll avoid overeating. On a practical level, this can help you cut calories from evening snacking. Walk away from the table when you've finished your main course at dinnertime. If you're still hungry after half an hour, go back and have seconds or eat your low-calorie dessert. If you're not hungry—and you probably won't be—you can save your dessert for later in the evening as a snack.

EMOTIONAL EATING

Do you eat only when you're hungry? Of course not—very few people do. Almost everyone succumbs to emotional eating sometimes. Whenever you feel stressed, angry, frustrated, anxious, sad, or just plain tired, it's perfectly normal to reach for comfort foods—and plenty of them. The problem isn't emotional eating, it's emotional *over*eating.

You don't have to fight off the perfectly normal desire to eat when you're under stress. Go ahead—but choose the right foods. This isn't always easy, of course, because most of us reach for exactly the wrong foods when we're eating emotionally. We want sugary, high-calorie foods such as cookies or chocolate, or we want high-fat, high-calorie snack foods such as potato chips.

You can satisfy your emotional need to eat without overloading on calories by sticking to low-calorie foods. Try choosing crispy, crunchy, low-calorie foods such as baby carrots, celery sticks, apples, frozen grapes, low-fat baked crackers, plain air-popped popcorn, or fat-free pretzels. If you want a sweet treat, try sugar-free gelatin or pudding, or make yourself a smoothie with low-fat yogurt and some frozen strawberries. Some calorie counters find that a high-protein snack helps them in times of stress. Try some low-fat cheese, some plain sliced turkey, a baked chicken leg, some low-fat yogurt, or even a peanut-butter sandwich. A bowl of hot soup is always very soothing and satisfying, plus hot liquids are helpful for cutting hunger pangs.

When you choose healthier foods, your emotional eating will at least be better for you. By making the choice to eat low-calorie foods, you're also controlling your emotional eating simply by being aware of it. The next time you find yourself eating emotionally, stop and think for a minute before you reach for the food. Ask yourself honestly why you're eating. If the answer is because you're upset or angry about something, you've taken the first step toward cutting back on your emotional overeating. Simply recognizing that you're eating from emotion, not hunger, is crucial. Learn to recognize emotional eating cues such as anger, loneliness, or feeling unappreciated or a little down. Once you realize why you're eating, you can refocus your energies into something more productive and healthier. Take a walk, work on a crafts project, have a bubble bath, enjoy a good book, call a friend, volunteer in your community—do something that makes you feel good without eating.

If you're prone to emotional overeating, learn to take care of yourself. If you tend to eat when you're overtired, for example, get more sleep—even if that means cutting back on other activities. Try to remove some stress from your life. That's not always easy, of course, but when you put your own emotional well-being higher on your priority list, you may find some ways.

And if you do end up eating a lot of high-calorie foods because you're feeling down or upset, don't make things worse by deciding your weight-loss efforts are hopeless. They're not. Learn from the experience and get yourself back on track as soon as you can. When you count calories and get regular exercise, your occasional lapses balance out in the long run.

YO-YO DIETING

How many times have you gone on a diet, lost weight, and then gone off the diet and gained it all back—and then some? If you're like most overweight people, this has happened more times than you want to admit. Doctors call this sort of up-and-down weight-loss weight cycling; dieters call it yo-yo dieting.

There are a lot of myths about weight cycling, but they turn out not to be true when you look at them more closely.

It's not true, for instance, that if you regain lost weight it will be harder to lose it again. Of course, you may be older by then, which does make it a little harder to lose weight, but the regained weight isn't somehow more resistant to dieting. There's also no evidence that weight cycling increases your risk of developing heart disease, high blood pressure, or diabetes.

The real question is, is it better to stay overweight or to have your weight go up and down? The answer is that losing weight is definitely healthier. There are no conclusive studies to show that weight cycling is harmful to the health of an obese person—but there are plenty of studies proving the health risks of obesity.

Once you learn to count calories, however, yo-yo dieting will be a thing of the past for you. You won't be constantly "going on a diet." Instead, you'll be eating a normal, balanced diet all the time. You'll be choosing the foods you like and even having the occasional rich dessert, while losing weight and keeping it off. You'll know how many calories you need to eat each day to meet your weight goals. Once you know how to choose the right foods and the right portion sizes, you won't need someone else's diet plan to tell you what to eat. You'll know for yourself.

PLATEAUS: WHEN WEIGHT LOSS STALLS

Plateaus—periods when your weight seems stuck and you just can't seem to start losing again—can be very frustrating. If you look closely and honestly at your calorie intake, however, you may well pin down the cause of your plateau. You're probably taking in more calories than you think. Are you really tracking all your calories accurately? Have you been forgetting some snacks? Are you underestimating the size of your portions? It's very easy to forget some calories and end up taking in more than you realize. Estimate your portions carefully and use your food diary and the calorie counter in this book to record your true intake.

If you really are taking in under 2,000 calories a day and you're still not losing weight, try increasing your activity level. As you'll learn in Chapter 4, exercise is a crucial element for weight loss. There's no better way to crash through a weight-loss plateau than to exercise more. The increased activity will jump-start your weight loss.

FINDING THE LOW-CALORIE ALTERNATIVE

By using some simple, tasty low-calorie alternatives to high-calorie foods, you can cut 250 calories from your daily intake without even noticing. Here are a few examples:

• Use low-fat margarine (about 50 calories per tablespoon) instead of butter (108 calories per tablespoon). Calories saved: 58. (Choose a margarine or spread that has no trans fats.)

• Use ketchup (16 calories per tablespoon), mustard (5 calories per tablespoon), or light mayonnaise (50 calories per tablespoon) instead of regular mayo (100 calories per tablespoon). Calories saved: between 50 and 95.

• Top your baked potato with 2 tablespoons fat-free sour cream (30 calories) instead of using 1 tablespoon butter (108 calories). Calories saved: 78.

• Use a low-calorie version of your favorite salad dressing instead of the full-calorie version. Calories saved: around 50 per tablespoon.

• Have broth-based soups such as chicken noodle (70 calories in half a cup) instead of cream-based soups such as cream of chicken (130 calories in half a cup). Calories saved: 60.

• Drink a diet soda (0 calories per 8 ounces) instead of the regular kind (100 calories per 8 ounces). Calories saved: 100.

• Instead of a chocolate milk shake (360 calories), make a smoothie with low-fat chocolate milk (160 calories). Calories saved: 200.

• Instead of a chicken breast with skin (300 calories), eat the breast without the skin (190 calories). Calories saved: 110.

With a little practice, you'll soon find plenty of satisfying alternatives to higher-calorie foods. The calorie charts in Chapter 6 will help you find lower-calorie choices. Table 3.1 on page 48 is a helpful quick guide for comparing higher-fat, higher-calorie foods to their lower-fat, lower-calorie alternatives.

Don't forget that smaller portions mean fewer calories. If you just can't give up cream of mushroom soup in favor of chicken broth, continue to enjoy it—but have a cup instead of a bowl. You can still treat yourself to a real chocolate shake every once in a while—just make it a small one instead of a giant one. And if you can't resist the big shake, make up for it by cutting calories somewhere else or exercising harder.

COOKING TO CUT CALORIES

How you cook your food makes a big difference in how many calories it contains. Deep-frying, for instance, adds a lot of calories from the frying oil and from any coating or batter you use. To save on calories while eating simple, delicious, and healthful meals, switch to some better cooking methods. Whenever possible, steam, broil, or bake— these methods don't add fat but do maximize the flavors of your foods. If you want to pan fry or sauté, you can cut

Table 3.1 Choosing the Low-Calorie Alternative

HIGHER-FAT FOOD	LOWER-FAT ALTERNATIVE
Dairy Products	
Whole milk	Low-fat (1%), reduced-fat (2%), or fat-free (skim) milk
Ice cream	Sorbet, sherbet, low-fat or fat-free frozen yogurt, low-fat ice cream, frozen fruit bar, frozen pudding bar
Whipped cream	Imitation whipped cream
Sour cream	Low-fat sour cream or plain low-fat yogurt
Cream cheese	Neufchâtel, light cream cheese, fat-free cream cheese
Cheese	Reduced-calorie cheese, low-calorie cheese, fat-free cheese
Regular (4%) cottage cheese	Low-fat (1%) or reduced-fat (2%) cottage cheese
Whole-milk mozzarella	Part-skim milk mozzarella
Whole-milk ricotta	Part-skim milk ricotta
Cereals, Grains, Pasta	
Ramen noodles	Rice or pasta
Pasta with white sauce (alfredo)	Pasta with red sauce (marinara)
Pasta with cheese sauce	Pasta with vegetables (primavera)
Granola	Bran flakes, crispy rice, grits, oatmeal, reduced-fat granola
Meat, Fish, Poultry	
Cold cuts or lunch meats	Low-fat cold cuts
Hot dogs	Low-fat hot dogs
Bacon or sausage	Canadian bacon or lean ham
Ground beef	Extra-lean ground round or ground turkey
Chicken or turkey with skin	Chicken or turkey without skin
Oil-packed tuna	Water-packed tuna
Beef chuck, rib, brisket	Beef round, loin
Pork spareribs	Pork tenderloin, lean smoked ham
Frozen breaded fish or fried fish	Baked, broiled, poached fish or shellfish
Frozen dinners	Reduced-fat frozen dinners
Pork sausage	Turkey sausage
Baked Goods	
Croissant	Hard roll
Doughnuts, muffins, scones, pastries, sweet rolls	English muffins, bagels, reduced-fat or fat-free muffins or scones
Cake (pound, chocolate, yellow	Cake (angel food, white, gingerbread)
Cookies	Graham crackers, gingersnaps, fig bars

Snacks and Sweets

Nuts	Dry-roasted nuts
Buttered popcorn	Air-popped light popcorn
Custards and puddings, gelatin	Skim-milk or sugar-free puddings, sugar-free flavored gelatin

Fats, Oils, Salad Dressings

Butter	Trans fat–free margarine or spread
Mayonnaise	Reduced-fat mayonnaise, mustard, ketchup
Regular salad dressings	Reduced-calorie or fat-free dressings, lemon juice, herb-flavored vinegar
Oils and shortening	Nonstick cooking spray, apple or prune puree in baked goods

the amount of butter or oil you need by using a no-stick frying pan (this makes cleanup easier too) or a nonstick cooking spray. You can also use a little chicken broth or wine instead of the fat.

Because meat is high in calories and vegetables are relatively low, try cooking dishes that combine the two, being sure to go heavy on the veggies and light on the meat. Try Chinese-style stir-fries—they're delicious and quick—or a pot of beef stew with lots of interesting different vegetables.

FINDING THE HIDDEN SUGAR

Hidden sugars are a real trap for unwary calorie counters. Take a look at Table 3.2 on page 50 and you'll see why—sweeteners of all sorts are high in calories. That means you have to watch out not just for plain white table sugar but also for brown sugar, molasses, maple syrup, honey, and other high-calorie sweeteners.

You also have to know how to read the package label to avoid the hidden sugar trap. Labels can be very misleading. When a box of breakfast cereal such as granola claims it has no sugar added, for instance, that doesn't mean the cereal has no sugar or that it's low in calories. The

Table 3.2 Calories in Sweeteners

SWEETENER	PORTION	CALORIES
Brown sugar	1 tablespoon	52
Brown sugar	1 cup	827
Corn syrup	1 tablespoon	60
Honey	1 tablespoon	64
Maple syrup	1 tablespoon	52
Molasses	1 tablespoon	53
Pancake syrup	¼ cup	200
Turbinado sugar	1 teaspoon	15
White table sugar (sucrose)	1 teaspoon	15
White table sugar	1 tablespoon	50
White table sugar	1 cup	774

cereal still has a fair amount of natural sugar, probably from the fruit that's in it. And granola is actually pretty high in calories—depending on the brand you choose, one small serving (about ½ cup) has well over 200 calories without the milk.

To find the hidden sugar, you have to know what to look for. Table 3.3 on page 51 gives you a list of nutritive sweeteners—or other words for added sugar. Always remember that sugar is sugar, whether it comes from white table sugar or supposedly more healthful sweeteners such as fruit-juice concentrate or honey.

To save the sugar calories, try no-calorie sweeteners instead. These sweeteners are extremely intense, which is why you get a lot of sweet taste from amounts so small that they have no or very few calories. Look for acesulfame K (Sweet One®, Swiss Sweet®), aspartame (Equal®, NutraSweet®), saccharin (no longer considered a cancer risk), or sucralose (Splenda®). Which sweetener you prefer is a matter of personal taste—try them to find the one you like. Read the package information carefully to find out how to use the sugar substitute for baking. If you're diabetic, discuss the use of sugar substitutes with your doctor.

Table 3.3 Other Names for Sugar	
Brown sugar	Invert sugar
Corn syrup	Lactose
Corn syrup solids	Maltose
Dextrose	Malt
Fructose	Mannitol
Fruit-juice concentrate	Molasses
Glucose	Sorbitol
High-fructose corn syrup	Sucrose (table sugar)
Honey	Xylitol

MEAL PLANNING FOR WEIGHT LOSS

It sounds impossible, but a good way to lose weight is to eat more. Instead of eating a main course and a dessert for dinner, try having a four-course meal. Start with a cup of vegetable soup, then move on to a big plate of salad greens with your favorite low-calorie dressing. Then have your main course—a baked chicken breast, for example. Instead of having just a small baked potato with it, have some steamed broccoli as well. By the time dessert comes around, you'll be too stuffed to want any. In fact, you may not have gotten through your main course.

By starting your meal with a satisfying cup of hot soup, you reduce your appetite—hot liquids have this effect quickly. By going on to a salad, you fill up with low-calorie but nutrient-rich, fiber-rich greens. Adding some broccoli to your main course adds only a handful of extra calories, but it gives you more to eat and enjoy and keeps you from feeling deprived by a small portion of the main dish. If you still have room for dessert after all that, you'll be satisfied with a much smaller portion. The end result? A very filling and enjoyable meal—and fewer calories.

Even if you can't take the time to prepare a four-course dinner every night, it's easy to have a salad or some soup before your lunch or dinner. You'll notice the difference in your reduced appetite for the main course. Your meal will also stick with you longer, keeping you from hunger pangs and between-meal snacks later on.

SNACK ATTACKS

Snacking on high-calorie, high-fat foods is the quickest way to pack on the pounds. In fact, those potato chips and late-night bowls of ice cream are probably one reason you're reading a book about weight loss.

The best way to avoid the calories from these foods is to remove them from your home. If there's a container of chocolate fudge ripple ice cream in your freezer, sooner or later you're going to eat it. Get rid of it instead. Ditto for all the other junk food in the house. If it's not there, you can't eat it. Your kids may complain, but is that stuff any better for them than it is for you? Teach your kids to snack on more healthful foods, such as fruit and cheese. If you want to treat the kids to some chips or some cookies, buy the smallest possible packages so the food will be eaten up quickly.

Getting rid of the junk food doesn't get rid of the urge to snack. When a snack attack strikes, give in—sensibly. Low-calorie snacks, such as fresh or dried fruit, celery sticks, popcorn, some low-fat cheese, or a cup of hot soup, satisfy your desire for a quick bite without adding a lot of calories.

When you snack, prepare a portion, put it on a plate, and put the rest of the food away. If you settle down in front of the TV with a whole container of a snack food, chances are you'll eat all of it. Too much of even a low-calorie snack adds up. Control your portion right from the start and you won't end up with too many calories.

DRINK UP!

The next time you feel like reaching for a cookie, try reaching for a glass of cold water or low-cal beverage instead. Whether you realize it or not, there's a good chance you're thirsty, not hungry, and drinking something will get rid of your food craving.

Nutritionists are unanimous that everyone should be drinking at least eight 8-ounce glasses of caffeine-free liquid every day—that's 64 ounces, or about 2 liters. As you'll realize when you start keeping a food diary, however, you're probably not drinking anywhere near that much. The liquids you do drink may be having the opposite effect of giving your body the water it needs. Beverages with caffeine in them—coffee, tea, colas, and other caffeinated sodas—have a diuretic effect. They make you produce more urine, which removes fluid from your system.

Successful calorie counters tend to be big drinkers. Water is the top choice—it's easy to get and it's free (if you drink perfectly good tap water instead of expensive designer water). Keep a sports bottle full of water handy at all times—on your desk, in your car, in your bag. Other good sources of low-calorie liquids are caffeine-free coffee, tea, and herbal teas. Caffeine-free diet sodas and flavored seltzers are also good choices. Caffeine-free diet iced tea, lemonade, and fruit drinks are fine, but watch out for fruit juice—it's very high in calories. To cut back on juice calories, try mixing just 2 ounces juice with 6 ounces water or plain seltzer. If you're sticking to plain water, toss in a few slices of lemon or lime for flavor.

ALCOHOLIC BEVERAGES

You can still enjoy a relaxing alcoholic beverage while counting calories, but choose carefully and drink in moderation. Most beers contain between 150 and 170 calories in a 12-ounce serving. Light beers have about 100 calories in 12 ounces. A 3.5-ounce glass of any kind of table wine has about 75 calories. There are about 100 calories in a jigger (1.5 ounces) of distilled spirits such as whiskey, vodka, or gin; sweetened creme liqueurs have more. Mixers such as orange juice or ice cream add more calories. And watch out for those bar snacks!

DINING OUT

Restaurant portions today are so large that you could get your entire day's worth of calories from just one meal. You don't have to give up on dining out, though. Some simple strategies will let you continue to count calories while enjoying a good meal cooked by someone else. The next time you eat out:

- Order an appetizer as your main course.

- Split an entree with someone else at the table.

- Ask your server if you can order a half-size portion.

- Eat only half your entree and ask for a doggie bag—you get to enjoy the meal twice.

- Order á la carte instead of going for the complete lunch or dinner.

- Have a cup of soup or salad as an appetizer.

- Ask the server to remove the bread basket after you've had a small portion.

- If you want dessert, split it with someone else at the table.

You can also select entrees that are lower in calories. Avoid rich sauces and anything deep-fried. Look for dishes that are steamed, poached, baked, roasted, grilled, stir-fried, or lightly sautéed. If you're in doubt, ask your server.

Try to avoid buffet restaurants—portion control gets very difficult. If the buffet is unavoidable, try to stick to lower-calorie choices, such as baked chicken, vegetables, and green salad. Be careful about salad bars too. It's very easy to load up a low-calorie green salad with lots of high-calorie extras and creamy dressing. Cole slaw, potato salad, pasta salad, and the like are surprisingly high in calories—take just a small amount.

If you're careful, you can even enjoy eating at fast-food restaurants. The most important thing to remember here is to say no when you're asked if you want to make your meal larger. Watch out for the combo meals as well—you could easily get more than a day's worth of calories from the special sandwich, large fries, and soft drink.

Good choices at fast-food restaurants include regular hamburgers, grilled chicken sandwiches, baked potatoes, and salads with low-fat dressing. If you can't resist the french fries (who can?), order the smallest portion.

PARTY TIME

Calorie counting can be a real challenge during the holidays and at parties. You're surrounded by food and by people urging you to eat it. Fortunately, you can enjoy yourself without going too far off your weight-loss program.

Start by being realistic. You're just not going to be losing any weight during the holiday season. A better goal would be not gaining any. You can hold the line with these simple strategies:

• If you know a big dinner is coming up, save some calories for it. Eat a good breakfast but go easy on snacks and lunch.

• Enjoy your favorite seasonal foods and skip the others. You can have a baked potato any day, but pumpkin pie only comes around at Thanksgiving.

• Skip the alcoholic beverages in favor of diet soda or seltzer. If you want a small amount of alcohol, try a wine spritzer.

• Dips and hors d'oeuvres can be very high in calories. Choose raw vegetables instead of chips and take just a small amount of dip. Limit the hors d'oeuvres you eat by sampling just one of each.

• At the buffet, take a small plate instead of a large one and fill it up—you'll feel like you're eating more. If you want seconds, go back for more salad or vegetables.

• If all the food is high in calories, make the best choices you can under the circumstances, keep your portions small, and enjoy. You can make up for the extra calories by cutting back a little over the next few days and working out more.

CUTTING CALORIES ON THE JOB

Watching your calories can be particularly difficult at your job. It's hard to resist the doughnuts and other sweet snacks coworkers bring in to share at break time. You might even be expected to bring them in yourself once in a while. It's also hard to avoid the food at office celebrations like birthdays and holidays. And on top of all that, you might have so many other personal things to do on your lunch hour that a fast-food restaurant is the only way you'll have time to eat.

There are some solutions to healthy eating on the job. When coworkers offer you high-calorie doughnuts or muffins, thank them and take one—only one. Eat only half of it—enough to be polite but not enough to throw your calorie count for the day out the window. (This will be much easier to do if you've followed the advice earlier in this chapter and eaten a good breakfast before you went to work.) And when it's your turn to bring breakfast, go ahead and buy those croissants for the gang. Just because you're counting calories doesn't mean they are.

Keep some high-quality snacks handy in your desk

drawer or bag so you have something to eat that doesn't come from the coffee cart or a vending machine. Choose foods that are easy to prepare or come in convenient packages—rice cakes, baked crackers, cheese slices, fresh fruit, carrot sticks. If you don't have easy access to a refrigerator or microwave during the workday, invest in an inexpensive insulated sandwich bag and a thermal container to keep foods cold or hot. Meal-replacement drinks and bars are very helpful for those busy days when you just don't have time for lunch.

QUIT SMOKING AND LOSE WEIGHT

Of all the things you can do to improve your health, quitting smoking is the most important—even more important than losing weight. But many people worry that if they give up cigarettes, they'll gain weight. In fact, some smokers do gain a few pounds when they quit, although very few gain a lot of weight. Smoking is much more harmful to your health than gaining a few pounds. It pays to quit.

Why do people gain weight when they give up smoking? As your body adjusts to the lack of nicotine, you might gain 3 to 5 pounds in water weight in the first week after you quit. You'll slowly lose it again over the next few weeks. The nicotine in tobacco also helps suppress your appetite. After the nicotine leaves your system, you may find yourself eating more. The solution here? Instead of reaching for a cigarette, reach for a crunchy carrot stick instead of a cookie. The longer or more you smoked, the more likely you are to gain weight, but even long-time heavy smokers don't usually gain more than 10 pounds in the year after they quit.

The secret to avoiding weight gain when you give up smoking is to improve your diet and start exercising more *before* you quit. You'll feel better and you'll be able to get through the difficult first few weeks without cigarettes more easily.

SHATTERING THE WEIGHT-LOSS MYTHS

An amazing number of weight-loss myths float around out there. Now that you know the importance of calorie counting, you know how wrong they are.

Here's one myth that's been around for years: Eating after 8 P.M. causes weight gain. The truth is that it doesn't matter what time of day you eat—it's how much you eat over the whole day and how much exercise you get.

Here's another myth: Foods like grapefruit, celery, and cabbage soup magically "burn" fat and make you lose weight. You know by now there's no magic or quick way to weight loss and that eating nothing but these foods for a few weeks is a very unhealthful way to lose weight.

You'll doubtless hear a lot of other weight-loss myths. Use your common sense and stick to your basic plan of cutting back on calories, eating a nutritious, well-balanced diet, exercising more, and losing weight slowly, steadily, and permanently.

Chapter Four
EXERCISE TO BURN CALORIES

Eat less, exercise more, and you'll lose weight faster than if you only cut calories. You'll also look better and feel better faster, and you'll be doing a lot to improve your long-term health.

Exercise is the secret ingredient of all successful calorie counters. When you cut your intake of calories and also increase your output of calories, you create a winning weight-loss combination. And if you know the exercise secret, you give yourself a lot of extra flexibility when you count your calories. If you have one of those days where extra calories just can't be avoided, you can make up the difference with some extra exercise over the next few days. In fact, if you're simply trying to keep ahead of the almost inevitable weight gain that comes with growing older, exercise alone might do the trick for you. Just increasing your daily activity level, assuming you keep your calorie intake to about 2,000 calories a day if you're a woman, can keep your weight steady as you age and even lead to some weight loss. To lose even a moderate amount of weight by exercise alone, however, you'd have to work out fairly hard for about an hour a day.

If you're also watching calories, however, you don't need to become a real gym rat to lose weight by increasing your activity level. You don't need to set foot in the gym at all. As you'll discover in this chapter, 30 minutes of moderate exercise a day is enough to speed up your weight loss if you also watch the calories. The exercise can be any activity you choose—even vacuuming the house counts.

BEYOND WEIGHT LOSS

The benefits of increased activity will help your health even if you don't lose a single pound. Here's what the latest scientific research says exercise can do for you:

• Lower your blood pressure if it's too high and help prevent high blood pressure if you're at risk.

• Improve your insulin sensitivity if you have adult-onset (Type 2) diabetes and help prevent diabetes if you're at risk.

• Improve your heart health and lower your risk of heart disease.

• Cut your risk of breast cancer sharply—by 40 percent or more—and cut your overall risk of cancer by about a third.

• Help keep you mentally sharp as you age and may help prevent Alzheimer's disease.

• Strengthen your bones and help prevent osteoporosis (thin, brittle bones that break easily) as you get older.

• Improve your balance and endurance and help prevent falls.

Exercise also improves how you look and feel. As your muscles firm up, your clothes fit better and you stand taller. You have more energy and endurance, you feel more alert in general, and you're less likely to feel a little depressed.

For calorie counters, one of the greatest benefits of ex-

ercise is that it helps control eating. You'll soon notice that
working out even a little cuts your appetite. It's a great way
to deal with food cravings—instead of reaching for a candy
bar, do something physical instead. Often just a few
minutes of any sort of exercise is enough to kill the craving.

The good news about exercise is that it helps everyone,
no matter how inactive you've been before and no matter
how old you are. In fact, 90-year-old women who start
lifting weights show amazing strength gains and improvement in their ability to get around on their own. If they can
do it, so can you. Even if you don't lose weight, adding
exercise to your life will still improve your health. Several
recent studies have shown that if you're fat and fit, you're
better off than if you're normal weight and out of shape.

The best news of all? Muscles are more metabolically
active than fat. In other words, the more muscles you have,
the quicker you burn the calories you take in—eight times
as fast. And after you work out, your body stays at a higher
metabolic rate for at least 30 to 60 minutes, even if you're
resting, so you continue to burn calories at a slightly higher
rate. Once you've achieved your weight goal, keep exercising and you'll find that because your metabolism now
runs a little faster, you can add some extra calories to your
daily level without regaining weight.

BEFORE YOU START

Exercise helps just about everyone lose weight and feel
better, but before you get started on an exercise program,
get yourself checked out by your doctor. This is particularly
important if you're over age 40, if you have been very
inactive, or if you have any sort of ongoing health problem,
such as high blood pressure, heart disease, diabetes, arthritis, back trouble, or anything else. Your doctor will tell you
if there are any medical restrictions on how much or what
sorts of exercise you can do. Chances are that as long as

you start slowly and don't overdo, almost any exercise will be fine.

To avoid injuries, do some basic stretching exercises at the start of any exercise session, and do some cool-down stretches when you're done. Pace yourself—never force yourself beyond your upper comfort level. Some minor muscle soreness after a workout is normal, but sharp or severe pain isn't. If you experience sudden or severe pain during your exercise, or if you feel faint or breathless, stop at once. You may have injured yourself or overdone your exercising. Check with your doctor if the pain continues or you don't feel better within a few minutes of stopping.

HOW MUCH EXERCISE?

Numerous studies have shown that 30 minutes of moderate exercise a day is all it takes to improve your health and help you lose weight. Those 30 minutes don't even have to be continuous—three 10-minute sessions are just as good as 30 straight minutes for getting the exercise edge. You might not be able to fit half an hour of uninterrupted exercise into your schedule, but just about anyone can manage 10 minutes here and there throughout the day. Although 30 minutes a day is ideal for seeing real improvement in your fitness, even 10 minutes a day will give you some benefit. If you can't manage 30 minutes every day, aim for every other day instead.

BURNING CALORIES

Look at Table 4.1 to see how various activities help you burn off calories. Just cleaning the house for half an hour will burn off 150 calories; going for a 30-minute walk at lunchtime will burn 130 calories. Combine the two and you've worked off 280 calories for the day.

Table 4.1 Calorie-Burning Activities

ACTIVITY	CALORIES BURNED IN			
	15 min.	30 min.	45 min.	60 min.
Aerobics, low-impact	135	270	405	540
Aerobics, high-impact	165	330	495	660
Bicycling, 6 mph	75	150	225	300
Bowling	25	50	75	100
Cleaning	75	150	225	300
Cooking	50	100	150	200
Cross-country skiing	145	290	435	580
Dancing (line)	65	130	195	260
Dancing (swing)	110	220	330	440
Downhill skiing	100	200	300	400
Gardening	90	180	270	360
Golf (walking)	45	90	135	180
Ice-skating	110	220	330	440
In-line skating	150	300	450	600
Jogging, 5 mph	185	370	555	740
Jumping rope	170	340	510	680
Martial arts	180	360	540	720
Racquetball	110	220	330	440
Rowing machine	150	300	450	600
Running, 8 mph	225	450	675	900
Sex (average pace)	25	50	75	100
Stairclimber	155	310	465	620
Swimming, 25 yds/min	130	260	390	520
Tennis	100	200	300	400
Walking, 3 mph	65	130	195	260
Water aerobics	70	140	210	280
Weight training	130	260	390	520
Yoga	70	140	210	280

Note: Figures are for 150-pound person.
Source: President's Council on Physical Fitness and Sports

Combine your 280 calories of exercise with the 250 calories you've cut from your diet, and you get 530 fewer calories for the day. At that rate, you'll lose a pound (3,500 calories) in exactly a week. You'll be feeling better and stronger overall—and the house will be cleaner!

Here's another exercise incentive for you: The heavier you are, the more calories you will burn as you exercise. That's because the estimates in Table 4.1 for the number of calories an activity uses are based on someone who weighs 150 pounds. If you're heavier than that, you have to move more weight, which means the activity will use even more calories.

Getting regular exercise is crucial for weight loss. Choose activities you enjoy—you'll be much more likely to stick with something that's fun. Set realistic goals. Just as your weight-loss goals should be achievable, so should your fitness goals. Aim for slow, steady gains in endurance, strength, and flexibility—but also intensify or lengthen your workout if it gets too easy. Track your progress in your daily food diary so you can see how your increased activity is helping your weight-loss program.

One of the best ways to help you stick to your fitness program is to have an exercise buddy or two. When you work out with someone else, you encourage each other and have someone with whom to share your progress. Many health clubs offer good deals when you join with a friend— take advantage of the opportunity.

WORKING IN YOUR EXERCISE

All the experts say that you should set aside a regular time for working out. That's fine in theory, but between work and family, it's often hard to find an extra 30 minutes a day for your exercise program, much less to do it at the same time every day. Experiment a little to find the best time of day for your exercise. Some people enjoy starting their day with an early-morning workout, but others prefer to wind down from the day by exercising on their way home. For others, a lunchtime workout or an evening session is most convenient. The one time to avoid exercise is near bedtime, because you might get so revved up that you won't be able to get to sleep. Go with what works best for you and your schedule—the important thing is to get your exercise whenever you can.

You may not be able to manage 30 straight minutes, but you can definitely find a lot of ways to work some additional activity into your day. Try parking at the far end of the lot when you get to work or go shopping and walking that extra little distance. Take the steps instead of the escalator or elevator for a couple of floors, or go up the stairs in your house a few extra times. Use your work breaks to take a short stroll or do a little stair-climbing—this will also keep you away from the doughnuts on the coffee cart or in the break room. You can even keep a light dumbbell in your office drawer and use it to exercise your arms while you're on the phone!

If you can't get away from your family for 30 minutes of exercise, try getting your family to join you instead. Go for a bike ride or a walk together, jump rope, or play tag in the backyard. If the rest of the family would really rather just watch TV, you can still join them—but do stretching or weight-training exercises or ride an exercise bike while you watch.

WALK IT OFF

Many authorities agree that of all the activities you can do to increase your calorie output, walking is top of the list. A recent study from Harvard Medical School showed that even a 10-minute daily stroll is enough to cut a woman's risk of heart disease nearly in half!

Walking has a lot of great advantages. It's inexpensive. You don't have to buy any fancy equipment—all you need is a comfortable pair of shoes with thick soles. You don't have to join a gym or take walking lessons. Walking is very safe. It has the lowest rate of injury of any form of exercise. It's also convenient. You can walk almost anywhere just about any time. Walking outdoors is always fun, because you can enjoy the scenery and get some fresh air and sunshine, but year-round climate-controlled indoor walking is as close and free as your nearest mall. In fact, you might be able to join a walking club at the mall. Some people find that a solitary walk is a great way to relax or think things over, but walking can also be a fun activity to share with a friend or get the whole family moving.

The Harvard study showed that it's the length of the walk, not how fast you go, that provides the heart benefit. In other words, it's better to walk longer at your natural pace than to push yourself to a faster pace for a shorter time.

If you've been very inactive, you might not be able to walk even 10 minutes nonstop. If you stick with it and walk just every other day, you'll be amazed at how quickly your endurance builds up. If you're like many people who take up walking, within a couple of months you could find yourself chugging along steadily every day for half an hour or longer.

As you begin your walking program, follow these tips:

• Wear comfortable, well-fitting walking shoes with socks. Dress for the weather.

• Choose a safe place to walk. Stay on the sidewalk whenever possible and watch out for traffic. If you walk at night, wear a reflective vest.

• Set a pace that lets you talk comfortably while you walk. If you can't carry on a conversation during your walk, you're walking too fast.

• Focus on your posture. Stand up straight, with your chin up and your shoulders slightly back.

• Swing your arms naturally and breathe deeply as you walk.

• If you want to listen to music through headphones, keep the volume down and watch out for traffic you might not hear.

Because a good walking pace still lets you talk comfortably, walking can be a very enjoyable social activity. Walk with your family and friends, or join a walking group in your community. By making regular dates to stroll with people whose company you enjoy, you'll be more likely to stick with your walking program.

WATER EXERCISE

Swimming and water exercise are an excellent way to get started on a fitness program. Swimming is enjoyable and very safe—you're unlikely to get injured. Water exercises are particularly helpful if you're very overweight or if you have joint problems such as arthritis. Because the water helps hold you up, you can exercise your joints without putting weight on them. Many community swimming programs, YMCAs, and local health clubs offer water exercise classes.

JOINING A HEALTH CLUB

Many calorie counters find that regular workouts at a health club help them stick to their exercise goals. But before you invest in a gym membership, consider these factors:

• **Location.** Is the club convenient to your home or workplace? If you have to go out of your way to get there, you may stop going at all.

• **Facilities.** Visit local health clubs to check out the facilities. The club should be spacious and clean; the locker rooms and showers should be clean, with no dirty towels piled in the corners.

• **Equipment.** The equipment should be modern and well maintained. Be sure there is enough of it; you don't want to have to wait or have time limits during busy periods.

• **Hours and class schedule.** Most clubs open early and stay open late, but make sure the club you're joining will be open at times that are convenient for you. Look for a club that offers a good mix of exercise classes, such as aerobics and yoga, at a variety of levels, and on a convenient schedule so you can find a class time that's good for you.

• **Atmosphere.** You should feel comfortable at the health club. If the gym caters to the local muscleheads and plays blaring music, it's probably not the right place for you. Look for friendly trainers and a relaxed atmosphere. When you visit, look for people in your age group or at your fitness level.

• **Cost.** Health club memberships can be costly. Before you sign up for an expensive year-long membership, ask for a day pass or trial membership to be sure you're happy with your choice. It's probably better to go with a month-to-month arrangement than a long-term contract. Some clubs offer free child care and extras such as towels, but some charge—be sure to read the fine print carefully.

Shop around to find the right gym. Be sure to visit at the busiest time of day—usually early morning or early evening. That's when you can see if the club gets uncomfortably crowded.

PERSONAL TRAINERS

A few sessions with a personal trainer can help you get your exercise program off to a really good start. If you're working with weights, it's important to have a trainer show you how to do the exercises safely and correctly. You also need someone to teach you how to use exercise machines and cardio equipment.

Often an introductory session or two with a personal trainer is part of your gym membership. You might have to pay for sessions after that, but once you've got the hang of things, you don't need to work with a trainer every time you go to the gym. An occasional session when you want to add more weight or different exercises to your routine could well be enough.

When choosing a trainer, watch him or her working with other clients. Is the trainer enthusiastic and supportive? Does the trainer always come on time? Look for a full-time professional trainer who is certified by a national organization such as the American Council on Exercise.

EXERCISE VIDEOS

Not everyone lives near a gym or wants to spend the money to join one. Or maybe you just prefer working out in the privacy and convenience of your own home. The solution for you may be exercise videos. Not all workout tapes are helpful or even safe, however. Here's what to look for:

- An experienced instructor (celebrity or otherwise).

- Warm-up and cool-down exercises in the workout.

- Alternatives or modifications to the main workout for people at a lower fitness level.

- Exercises that include stretching, aerobics, and strength.

- If special equipment is needed, it should be inexpensive, sturdy, and available anywhere, not just from the video producer.

One of the fun things about videos is that there are a lot of good ones available. You can find a good selection at any video rental store or at your public library. Before you try doing the workout, though, watch the tape all the way through to make sure it meets the requirements listed and to be sure you're up to it. Once you've found a few tapes you like, swap them with friends to keep your workouts interesting.

Chapter Five

CALORIE COUNTING AND POPULAR DIET PLANS

When you look carefully at just about any of the many popular diet plans, you'll realize that they all come back to the same simple idea: calorie counting. It may be disguised by a special way of keeping track of the calories, or it may be disguised by telling you to eat only the foods the diet plan sells you, or it may be disguised in soy shakes and protein bars, but in the end, what you're doing on any plan is losing weight by cutting the number of calories you take in every day.

Cutting calories on your own can be difficult, even when you understand the concepts. Many dieters find that following a diet plan in a book helps them move at their own pace in privacy. Others find that participating in a structured weight-loss program that provides not only a basic diet concept but also support groups and personalized advice can be very, very helpful. This is especially true for people who have repeatedly tried to lose weight or who have lost weight and then gained it back.

Some of the popular diet plans are great. They provide well-balanced, tasty meal plans, teach you about good nutrition and portion control, remind you to exercise, and even make it a little simpler to track your calories. Because these plans help you make permanent lifestyle changes, they help you lose weight and keep it off.

Unfortunately, just because a diet plan is popular doesn't mean it's good. Choose the wrong plan and you won't be able to stick with it. You might even do real harm to your health.

With a little knowledge and some common sense, you can easily select a weight-loss program that will work for you.

CHOOSING THE RIGHT PROGRAM

As you can tell from the weight-loss section of any bookstore, all those ads on television, and all those products on the supermarket shelves, there are a lot of different diet plans out there. To find a plan that will work for you, here's what to look for:

• **Safety.** The diet plan should be safe and realistic—it should aim for slow, steady weight loss of 1 to 2 pounds a week. That means the diet should allow for anywhere from 1,200 to 1,800 calories a day.

• **Good nutrition.** A safe diet is low in calories but high in nutrition. The diet plan should provide you with the recommended daily allowance (RDA) of vitamins and minerals every day and should have at least 60 grams (8 ounces) of protein and 150 grams of carbohydrates daily.

• **Variety and flexibility.** A diet that restricts or forbids large groups of foods is too limiting to stick with for long and may not be providing adequate nutrition. Select a diet plan that provides a variety of foods and is flexible enough to adapt to your personal likes and dislikes.

• **Real food.** Prepackaged foods, shakes, and meal replacement bars can be good aids to weight loss, but you have to live in the real world. Look for a program that also teaches you how to prepare your own healthful foods, control your portions, and eat out safely.

• **Lifestyle changes.** A good diet plan goes on for more than just two weeks. It helps you make permanent lifestyle changes that let you achieve your weight goal and stay there—that means a plan that promotes overall healthy eating and exercise.

STRUCTURED DIET PLANS

About 50 million Americans a year sign up for some sort of structured weight-loss program. It's a big business, and there are a lot of for-profit companies that will gladly take your money to help you slim down. Companies such as Weight Watchers®, for example, have been doing a great job at a reasonable fee for many years. But before you sign up for a structured diet plan, be sure you really understand what the plan offers and what the costs will be. (The details of the various plans will be discussed later in this chapter.) Don't be taken in by ads that show someone who lost 150 pounds on that particular plan. Somewhere in that ad might be some fine print that says "Results not typical." Look carefully at the plan before you sign up. At a minimum, a good structured diet plan offers:

• Realistic weight and fitness goals

• Adequate calories, good nutrition, and a variety of foods

• Individualized assessments and counseling with a trained professional

• A convenient schedule, if the plan offers meetings and classes

• Online chats and online or phone counseling if you prefer or can't get to in-person meetings

• Follow-up and maintenance plans once you meet your weight-loss goal

• An itemized list of fees and costs

If you're considering a plan that offers prepackaged foods or special mixes and bars, check out the prices and availability. Ask how much is included in the basic fee and how much costs extra.

Before you sign a contract with a commercial diet plan, ask some final questions.

• How many people who sign up for the program actually complete it?

• On average, how much weight do they lose?

• What are the health risks and side effects of the plan?

• Is there a trial membership or cancellation period so you can be sure the plan is right for you?

Be sure you understand which services are part of the basic plan and which will cost more—and read the fine print.

SUPPORT GROUPS FOR WEIGHT LOSS

No matter how you decide to diet, it will be easier if you have some support from people who understand how difficult weight loss can be. Support is part of the deal with many commercial diet plans, but if you're on your own (and even if you're not), you may want to find some help in your community. An excellent organization for dieters is TOPS® (Take Off Pounds Sensibly). A nonprofit, noncommercial organization with no fees beyond the very modest membership fee, TOPS® is very accessible. Chapters provide lively meetings, presentations, workshops, incentives and support, and lots of helpful information. The organization does not promote any particular diet plan or products. Although TOPS® does suggest the exchange list program developed by the American Diabetes Association (discussed later in this chapter), the organization recommends that you work with your own doctor or nutritionist to set your weight-loss and fitness goals. TOPS® then helps you stick with your plan by providing support, recognition, encouragement, education, and friendship.

There are over 9,000 TOPS® chapters nationwide. To find a chapter near you, call (800) 932-8677 or go to *www.tops.org.*

Overeaters Anonymous (OA) is a 12-step program for compulsive overeaters. The OA program helps you address the physical, emotional, and spiritual aspects of compulsive overeating. Like TOPS, OA is not a diet plan—it is a support group for people with a common problem. There are thousands of OA groups nationwide. To find one near you, contact:

Overeaters Anonymous
PO Box 44020
Rio Rancho, NM 87174
(505) 891-2664
www.overeatersanonymous.org

DUMB DIETS

Can you really melt fat away while you sleep? Can you really lose 10 pounds in just a week? Should you follow a diet just because a Hollywood celebrity recommends it?

Fad diets, crash diets, magic supplement diets—you know by now that they won't work. All those claims that you can lose weight effortlessly are so much nonsense. You actually might lose a few pounds at the start, but it will be at the price of hunger and bad nutrition—and you will almost certainly gain the weight back as soon as you go off the diet. The basic rule of thumb here is that the faster you lose the weight, the faster you'll put it back on.

Even so, some dumb diets are still popular, no matter how often medical experts point out that these diets are unsafe. When you take a closer look at these diets, they all turn out to restrict your caloric intake. The popular cabbage soup diet, for instance, has you spend two weeks eating little else but a soup made of cabbage and other vegetables. You also eat, according to a strict schedule, some fruits and vegetables and occasional protein dishes, such as grilled fish or yogurt. You'll lose weight, but only because this diet plan is highly restrictive and gives you 1,200 calories a day at most. More than a couple weeks on this diet would lead to serious nutritional deficiencies, to say nothing of the effect of all that cabbage on your digestion. Despite the claims, there is nothing in cabbage that helps you "burn fat" away. Any weight loss comes only from the restricted calories.

Another popular area for diet fads is food combining. These diets claim that by eliminating some foods and eating or not eating other foods only in certain combinations or at certain times, you'll lose weight faster. Not only that, some say you'll "eliminate toxins," whatever that means, from your body. These plans work in the short run because they make choosing your food very complicated. You'll end up eating less as you eliminate some foods and try to follow the complex directions for eating the other foods at the right time and in the right combination. In the long run, however, these diets are so complicated and nutritionally imbalanced that it's almost impossible to stick to them.

There are many, many other fad diets that use some sort of gimmick. The grapefruit diet, for instance, has you eating little else. In the end, most of these fad diets have little scientific basis. Many come down to weight loss by a diet that is, for whatever reason, way too low in calories and nutrition, so stay away.

DIETS THAT WORK

For a diet plan to work, it needs to help you control your daily calories in a safe, sensible, and flexible way that fits into your lifestyle. Everyone's different, of course, which is why a diet plan that works well for one person may not be the right approach for another. Use the following descriptions to help you find the diet program that might work best for you.

Weight Watchers®

Weight Watchers® is probably the most successful diet program ever, because the sensible approach it takes to calorie counting is easy to follow and works in the real world. Rather than have you track your daily calories, Weight Watchers® has developed a simplified system that assigns points instead of calorie counts to your food. So, instead of aiming for anywhere between 1,200 and 1,800 calories a day, Weight Watchers® has you aim for anywhere between 18 and 35 points a day, depending on your weight. It works out to the same thing in the end—fewer calories. Common foods are assigned points by Weight Watchers® based on an analysis of their fat, fiber, and calorie content; lists are provided to Weight Watchers® participants as part of their membership.

Because foods that are high in fiber are generally very low in fat and calories, some foods, such as broccoli and lettuce, have 0 or only 1 point. Foods that are high in fat and calories are high in points.

Your daily points are divided into five categories—complex carbohydrates, protein, dairy products, fruits and vegetables, and fats. The program recommends point ranges within each category, such as 6 to 9 points from complex carbohydrates. If that number sounds vaguely familiar, check back to the discussion of the food pyramid in Chapter 2. The Weight Watchers® program is based in large part on the servings and portion sizes of the food pyramid—a very sensible and effective approach to weight management.

The Weight Watchers® program offers a lot of flexibility. As long as you stay within your points for the day, you can distribute them pretty much any way you want. Of course, the program encourages you to spread your points out in a healthy and well-balanced way within the recommended categories—you're not supposed to blow them all on potato chips and doughnuts. Though there aren't any forbidden foods, portion control is strongly emphasized, and the portions per point are small. A 1-point portion of orange juice, for instance, is just 4 ounces, a 1-point portion of cottage cheese is 3 ounces, and a single baked chicken drumstick without the skin counts as 1 point.

Once you understand the point system and get used to the portion sizes, you'll find that there are plenty of enjoyable 1-point and 0-point foods and snacks to fill up on. You can also "bank" some points if you know a big event or holiday is coming up.

The costs for joining Weight Watchers and attending meetings are very reasonable. The program offers a lot of group and individual support and strongly recommends exercise—in fact, you "earn" points for working out. To help you stick to the points program, Weight Watchers® offers a wide range of food products with the points already calculated, including a full line of frozen entrees, meals, and desserts. The Weight Watchers® point system is so popular that many food manufacturers list the points per portion on food labels.

Food Exchange Lists

By using a meal plan and food exchange lists, you can design your own weight-control diet. Food exchange lists such as those developed by the American Dietetic Association and the American Diabetes Association are actually very simplified forms of calorie counting. These lists were developed originally to help people with diabetes eat a healthy and varied diet and also lose weight if they need to, but they work well for anyone who wants to lose weight.

The basic concept of food exchange lists is that foods can be grouped into just a handful of basic categories. Within each category, a serving of any one food has about the same amounts of carbohydrates, protein, fat, and calories as any other food on that list. You can exchange, or swap, one food on the list for another. Within the starches in the carbohydrate group, for instance, 1 slice of whole-wheat bread is the equivalent of half an English muffin. So, you could trade one for the other at breakfast and count it as one starch portion, because each portion contains 15 grams of carbohydrate and 80 calories. Or, you could have the whole English muffin and count it as 2 starch portions. Likewise, in the fruits category, you can exchange 3 ounces of grapes for 1 cup of cantaloupe cubes or 1 small banana, because each portion contains 15 grams of carbohydrate and 60 calories.

The number of portions—and calories—you select each day from each exchange list category is based on your own individual needs. You work with your doctor or nutritionist to decide what's best for you and then figure out how many portions you need to have from each list. Because the exchange lists give you a lot of flexibility, you can choose your favorite foods within each category. If you get tired of a particular food, you can easily swap it for something more interesting.

Exchange lists can get fairly complex, but the basic concept isn't that hard. All your foods are divided into three basic groups: carbohydrates, meat and meat substitutes (beans and peas), and fat. Within the carbohydrate group, foods are divided into starches (bread, pasta, rice, and similar foods), fruit, milk, vegetables, and other carbohydrates such as jam and baked goods. Within the meat group, foods are divided into very lean, lean, medium-fat, and high-fat foods. Within the fat group are butter, oils, and shortenings as well as high-fat foods such as nuts and cream cheese. In the free foods category are foods such as beef bouillon and sugar-free gelatin that can be eaten as often as you like.

In the carbohydrate group, each starch portion has 80 calories, each fruit portion has 60 calories, each dairy portion has between 90 and 150 calories, and each vegetable portion has 25 calories. Meat and meat substitute portions range from 35 to 100 calories, and each fat portion has 45 calories.

Inexpensive publications from the American Diabetes Association and other organizations explain the exchange program and provide detailed food lists with portion sizes. To follow the program, you'll need to keep a food diary to track your portions and swaps, and the system won't work for you unless you are very careful about portion control. The portions for each individual food are small. When you're swapping one food for another, you need to be sure you're using the equivalent portion. Once you get the hang of it, though, exchange lists are fairly easy to use, and they give you plenty of choices. Because the system is now widely used, many food manufacturers now put the exchange points and portion sizes right on food labels.

For more information and publications about food exchange lists, contact:

American Diabetes Association
1701 North Beauregard Street
Alexandria, VA 22311
(800) 342-2383
www.diabetes.org

Calorie-Counting with Jenny Craig®

The Jenny Craig® program counts calories outright—no disguises here. That means less work for you, because the program provides you with detailed meal plans and prepared foods for all your meals. The Jenny Craig® program provides balanced nutrition and works well, but between the membership fee and the cost of the foods, it can be pricey.

Based on your weight-loss goals and general health, a Jenny Craig® consultant helps you choose between the 1,200-calorie and 1,500-calorie daily plan. Your goal is weight loss of 1 to 2 pounds a week; if you start losing faster, you'll be advised to eat more to keep your weight loss slow and steady. Until you lose half your extra weight, you'll be eating Jenny Craig® prepared foods for all your meals; you provide only a few extras such as nonfat milk and vegetables. The calorie counting is done for you. By eating only the prepared foods and specific amounts of additional foods, you get a better idea of what healthful portions and balanced nutrition are all about. Once your weight loss is well established, you work with your consultant to gradually add more of your own foods and eat less of the Jenny Craig® prepared foods. At this point the program teaches you how to control your calories by using the exchange list system described earlier.

Overall, the Jenny Craig® program offers sensible weight loss through calorie counting. The foods are nutritious and varied, and they're delivered right to your door. Some people can have trouble with the transition to the "real" world from eating only the prepared foods and following the meal plan. Once you have to make your own choices and control your own portions, it's possible to start overdoing on the calories again. Classes, meetings, and individual counseling sessions (by phone or online if you don't live near a Jenny Craig® Centre) are part of the Jenny Craig® program, however, and these help you stick with the plan and make the transition.

The same basic idea of providing you with calorie-controlled meals is behind other popular structured diet plans such as NutriSystem® and Diet Center®. These plans offer prepared foods based on a reduced-calorie diet, nutritional advice, personal counseling, and exercise advice. *Nutrisystem.com* is online for people who prefer privacy or who don't live near a meeting place.

Shake It Off with Slim•Fast®

The Slim•Fast® plan is a variation on the prepared meal approach. This plan recommends at least 1,200 calories a day and warns you not to use Slim•Fast® products as your only source of nutrition. To get 1,200 calories a day on the plan, you eat a Slim•Fast® shake or Slim•Fast® Meal On-The-Go bar to replace your usual breakfast and another to replace lunch. Both meal replacers contain 220 calories; your remaining calories come from a mid-morning and mid-afternoon low-calorie snack, such as fruit, and from a sensible dinner. The Slim•Fast® products are widely sold in supermarkets and health stores—you don't have to join a program or purchase your shakes and bars directly from the company. You're on your own when it comes to planning your snacks and sensible evening meal, although the free Slim•Fast® club provides some online guidance.

The shakes and bars are tasty, low in fat, and fortified with vitamins and minerals. They're very helpful for people on the go as a way to grab a convenient and satisfying low-calorie meal without resorting to a fast-food restaurant or skipping a meal. Because they all contain 220 calories, they help take some of the guesswork and tracking out of calorie-counting. The Slim•Fast® approach works for some people, particularly if they have busy schedules and can't take the time to prepare calorie-controlled meals three times a day. All those sweet shakes and bars can get monotonous, however, and the program is hard to stick with for more than a couple of weeks.

Low-Carb Calories

Made famous by the best-selling book *Dr. Atkins' New Diet Revolution*, low-carbohydrate dieting is the basic principle found in many other popular diet books, including *Sugar*

Busters by Leighton Steward and others, *Protein Power* by Michael and Mary Eades, and *The Carbohydrate Addict's Diet* by Richard and Rachel Heller. Although all these authors have impressive credentials as medical doctors or researchers, their work is very controversial. To understand why, you need to understand a little about how your metabolism works.

When you eat carbohydrates (sugary or starchy foods), the food is broken down into glucose ("blood sugar"), which provides energy for the cells of your body. The glucose is carried into your cells by the hormone insulin. The theory behind low-carbohydrate dieting is that eating large amounts of carbohydrates stimulates your body to produce excess insulin. The insulin very efficiently stores the extra carbohydrates by converting them into fat. If you eat only small amounts of carbohydrates, however, your body won't produce much insulin in response, and you won't have excess glucose in your blood to be converted into fat. In addition, if you're overweight and reduce your carbohydrate intake to a bare minimum, your body will use your stored fat for energy and you'll lose weight.

The logic behind low-carbohydrate dieting makes sense, but the diets upset the more traditional diet researchers. That's because low-carb dieting cuts out a lot of fruits, grains, and starchy vegetables such as potatoes. It also cuts many dairy products, such as milk, but allows high-fat foods, such as red meat, eggs, nuts, butter, cheese, and vegetable oils. This approach goes very much against the received nutritional wisdom that no more than 30 percent of your daily calories should come from fat.

Low-carbohydrate dieting works for a lot of people, however. They don't have to count calories, they lose weight slowly and steadily, and they don't get hungry. As a bonus, their cholesterol levels and blood sugar numbers usually improve as well.

It's hard to believe that you could lose weight on a diet that doesn't have you count your calories in some way, but it makes sense when you look at the diets more closely. Low-carbohydrate dieting eliminates or sharply reduces refined carbohydrates from your diet—no more cookies, snack foods, potato chips, bread, pasta, sugar, and similar foods. Their place in your diet is taken by unlimited amounts of low-carbohydrate, low-calorie vegetables such as salad greens and broccoli. When you cut the carbs, you're automatically cutting calories and improving your nutrition, because you're substituting healthy vegetables for processed foods such as french fries.

What about all that high-fat, calorically dense meat and other protein foods on a low-carb diet? Precisely because these foods contain fat and a lot of calories, they're very satisfying. A relatively small amount of steak or cheese, for example, fills you up more than a larger amount of pasta in a low-fat sauce and keeps you from getting hungry for longer. The end result is actually smaller meals and less between-meal eating. People on low-carbohydrate diets eat fewer calories without noticing, because they don't get as hungry. As for the fat content of the meals, the connection between saturated fat in the diet and high cholesterol and clogged heart arteries actually isn't all that clear. A lot of other factors probably play as big a role or an even bigger one.

After you've achieved your weight goals on a low-carbohydrate diet, you can gradually start adding high-quality carbohydrates (no junk foods allowed) back into your diet. At that point most people on a low-carb diet can eat anywhere from 50 to 100 grams of carbohydrates a day without gaining back any weight. To help keep your carbohydrate grams down and satisfy cravings for sweets, Atkins and other manufacturers offer a variety of low-carbohydrate bars, shake mixes, and other foods.

In general, low-carbohydrate eating plans don't have you restrict your portions or count calories. Instead, you choose your foods according to the general principles, which in turn means you end up eating fewer calories simply because you're not as hungry. Weight loss follows, because on average low-carb dieters eat anywhere from 250 to 1,000 fewer calories a day—without counting.

Zone in on Calories

In his best-selling book *Enter the Zone*, author Barry Sears, Ph.D., created a modified version of low-carbohydrate dieting. The Zone plan allows more carbohydrates than the other diets and probably ends up giving you fewer calories. On the Zone diet, 40 percent of your daily calories come from carbohydrates, 30 percent come from protein, and 30 percent come from fat. You can eat up to 250 grams a day of carbohydrates, but only from high-quality sources such as whole grains, fresh fruit, and leafy vegetables.

On the Zone plan, you don't count calories for each category, you count "blocks." A block is quite small—a single protein block, for example, is just 7 grams, or about 1 to 1.5 ounces of cooked meat, poultry, or fish, which is equal to about 28 calories. Depending on your body weight, your daily block totals would come to around 11 protein blocks, 11 carbohydrate blocks, and 11 fat blocks. The Zone blocks are carefully balanced to give you a nutrient-dense but low-calorie diet. When you add up all the blocks, the Zone diet works out to only about 1,200 calories a day. That's on the low side for weight loss and you're likely to be hungry between meals, but you will be getting well-balanced and varied meals if you follow the plan.

Very-Low-Calorie Diets

For some people, a very-low-calorie diet (VLCD) used under medical supervision is an effective way to lose weight. In general, these diets are appropriate only for people who need to lose 50 pounds or more or whose BMI is 30 or more.

Very-low-calorie diet plans such as Optifast®, Medifast®, HMR®, and the Cambridge Diet® replace all your food with special shakes, bars, and other products that limit your calories to anywhere from 500 to 1,200 a day. These programs are available only through doctors and medical centers with weight-loss clinics. You can't use the products on your own—you must be under medical supervision.

Before you go on a VLCD, you must have a complete medical workup; once you're on the program, you must see your doctor often for evaluations. Very-low-calorie diets are generally safe for people who are seriously overweight, but problems such as irregular heartbeat can develop—your doctor needs to keep an eye on your health. You also work with a registered dietitian to learn healthy eating habits and increase your exercise level. Some programs offer weight-loss drugs to their patients, but the medications aren't required. The programs also offer counseling, meetings, and support groups to help you cope.

The idea behind a very-low-calorie diet is to help you make a complete break with your past unhealthful eating patterns and then relearn a better way to eat. This radical approach doesn't work for everybody, but the programs have a fairly good track record for helping their patients lose weight and keep it off.

Between the cost of enrolling in the program, seeing your doctor often, and buying the special foods, these diets can be costly. Most people go on a VLCD because it's medically necessary, however, so your health insurance may cover some or all of the expenses.

Counting Fat Calories with Ornish and Pritikin

Extremely low-fat diets, with only 10 to 15 percent of your calories coming from fat, are designed for people with heart disease caused by clogged arteries. These diets aren't meant as weight-loss programs, but most people who follow them to improve their heart health also end up losing weight.

The two leading proponents of very low-fat diets are the late Nathan Pritikin, M.D., and Dean Ornish, M.D., founders of the Pritikin Center. The diets are described in popular books such as *The Pritikin Weight Loss Breakthrough* by Robert Pritikin, M.D., and *Eat More, Weigh Less* by Dean Ornish. In general, the Pritikin and Ornish diets are almost vegetarian. Both emphasize lots of whole grains, fruits, and vegetables, and practically eliminate animal protein, fat, and processed carbohydrates. Both diets average about 1,800 calories a day. At that rate, anyone who is overweight will lose weight.

The Pritikin and Ornish diet have been shown to help people with heart disease, but it's not clear if the diets actually will keep you from getting heart disease to begin with. Both diet programs also emphasize exercise and relaxation techniques, so it's also unclear how much of a role the very low fat content of each diet plays.

In general, the Pritikin and Ornish diets are low in calories. The Pritikin program doesn't count calories outright. Instead, you combine large portions of foods that are low in calories—whole grains or vegetables, for instance—with small portions of high-calorie foods such as olive oil or nuts. The Ornish program doesn't count calories either, but because it is essentially vegetarian and eliminates almost all fat, meat, and high-calorie foods, the foods that are allowed are naturally low in calories. You can eat your fill and you still probably won't exceed 1,800 calories a day.

It's possible to be creative within the food limits of these diets, but at bottom they are very restrictive. Many people find it very difficult to stick with a program that allows so few food choices and requires such careful preparation. Among other problems, it's very hard to eat out when following these diets, and you do need to take dietary supplements to be sure you're getting enough vitamins and minerals. It's also not clear what the long-term effects of a diet so low in fat might be. There's a lot of evidence to show that certain fats, such as fish oil and olive oil, help prevent some kinds of cancer and even improve heart health.

If you have heart disease, discuss the Pritikin and Ornish plans with your doctor before you try them. If your heart is healthy and you're overweight, consider other less extreme weight-loss programs first. If you'd still like to try a very-low-fat diet, discuss your plans with your doctor before doing so.

Chapter Six
CALORIE COUNTS FOR COMMON FOODS

The extensive charts that follow give you calorie counts and portions for over 2,500 common foods. The charts also provide the amounts of fat, protein, carbohydrates, and cholesterol in the foods. Where the information is available, an additional column lists added sugar; this number is part of, not in addition to, the total carbohydrate count. Information about added sugars is not required by federal regulations and it is often not provided by food manufacturers and restaurants. In such cases, the column is left blank, but it is still possible that the food contains added sugars. Sometimes other details about a food, such as the carbohydrate content, are not available, usually because the food contains the nutrient in only small amounts. In such cases the column is left blank.

The information in these charts comes from the U.S. Department of Agriculture and from food manufacturers and restaurants. It's as accurate and up-to-date as possible. Food manufacturers and restaurants sometimes reformulate their products, however, and some of the information may change slightly over time. Food producers and restaurants also vary their offerings, adding new products and removing old ones. Every effort has been made to include currently available products.

The portion sizes listed in these charts are based on the standard portions used by nutritionists or on the serving size provided by the food manufacturer. In general, these portions are smaller than what most people actually eat. When counting how many calories you will take in from eating a particular food, read the chart in this book or the food label carefully and be aware of the portion size.

Calorie counters should remember these benchmark numbers: There are 4 calories in a gram of carbohydrate or protein and 9 calories in a gram of fat. There are 3,500 calories in 1 pound of fat. Cutting your calories by 250 to 500 a day will lead to safe, steady weight loss.

Table 6.1 Calorie Counts

Food	Portion	Calories	Fat	Protein	Carb	Sugar	Chol
ALCOHOLIC BEVERAGES							
BEER AND ALE							
ale, Ballantine Pale	12 fl oz	186					
ale, Bass	12 fl oz	130					
ale, Genesee Cream	12 fl oz	154					
beer, Amstel Light	12 fl oz	102					
beer, Anchor Steam	12 fl oz	207					
beer, Beck's	12 fl oz	151					
beer, Bud Dry	12 fl oz	130	0.0	1.1	8.2	0.0	0
beer, Bud Ice	12 fl oz	148	0.0	1.3	9.2	0.0	0
beer, Bud Ice Light	12 fl oz	96	0.0	0.8	3.5	0.0	0
beer, Bud Light	12 fl oz	110	0.0	0.9	6.6	0.0	0
beer, Budweiser	12 fl oz	147	0.0	1.2	11.4	0.0	0
beer, Busch	12 fl oz	143	0.0	1.1	10.9	0.0	0
beer, Busch Ice	12 fl oz	169	0.0	1.3	12.8	0.0	0
beer, Busch Light	12 fl oz	110	0.0	0.8	6.7	0.0	0
beer, Coors	12 fl oz	137					
beer, Coors Light	12 fl oz	105					
beer, Genesee	12 fl oz	151					
beer, Genesee Light	12 fl oz	95					
beer, Heineken Lager	12 fl oz	165					
beer, Heineken Special Dark	12 fl oz	168					
beer, High Life	12 fl oz	143	0.0	1.0	13.1	0.0	0
beer, High Life Ice	12 fl oz	156	0.0	1.1	11.0	0.0	0
beer, High Life Light	12 fl oz	110	0.0	1.0	7.0	0.0	0
beer, Icehouse	12 fl oz	132	0.0	1.2	8.7	0.0	0
beer, King Cobra	12 fl oz	177	0.0	1.7	14.1	0.0	0

Food	Portion	Calories	Fat	Protein	Carb	Sugar	Chol
beer, Kirin	12 fl oz	186					
beer, Kronenbourg	12 fl oz	151					
beer, Lowenbrau Dark	12 fl oz	158	0.0	1.4	14.3	0.0	0
beer, Meisterbrau	12 fl oz	128	0.0	1.0	11.4	0.0	0
beer, Meisterbrau Light	12 fl oz	103	0.0	0.9	4.8	0.0	0
beer, Michelob	12 fl oz	157	0.0	1.3	13.5	0.0	0
beer, Michelob Classic Dark	12 fl oz	163	0.0	1.5	14.8	0.0	0
beer, Michelob Dry	12 fl oz	130	0.0	1.2	7.9	0.0	0
beer, Michelob Golden Draft	12 fl oz	151	0.0	1.6	13.1	0.0	0
beer, Michelob Golden Draft Light	12 fl oz	110	0.0	1.0	6.7	0.0	0
beer, Michelob Light	12 fl oz	134	0.0	1.0	11.5	0.0	0
beer, Michelob malt	12 fl oz	160	0.0	1.4	9.8	0.0	0
beer, Miller	12 fl oz	150	0.0	1.1	13.2	0.0	0
beer, Miller Lite	12 fl oz	96	0.0	0.9	3.2	0.0	0
beer, Miller Lite Ice	12 fl oz	113	0.0	0.9	4.0	0.0	0
beer, Milwaukee's Best	12 fl oz	128	0.0	0.9	11.4	0.0	0
beer, Milwaukee's Best Ice	12 fl oz	135	0.0	0.9	9.6	0.0	0
beer, Milwaukee's Best Light	12 fl oz	98	0.0	0.8	3.5	0.0	0
beer, Molson's	12 fl oz	151					
beer, Molson's Light	12 fl oz	81					
beer, Pabst Blue Ribbon	12 fl oz	151					
beer, Red Dog	12 fl oz	147	0.0	0.7	14.1	0.0	0
beer, Rolling Rock	12 fl oz	140					

Food	Portion	Calories	Fat	Protein	Carb	Sugar	Chol
beer, Samuel Adams	12 fl oz	175					
beer, Schaefer	12 fl oz	140					
beer, Schlitz	12 fl oz	144					
beer, Stroh's	12 fl oz	144					
malt beverage, O'Doul's	12 fl oz	70	0.0	0.7	14.0	0.0	0
malt beverage, Sharp's	12 fl oz	58	0.0	0.4	12.1	0.0	0
malt liquor, Colt 45	12 fl oz	158					
malt liquor, Schlitz	12 fl oz	182					
WINE AND LIQUOR							
bloody mary	5 fl oz	148	0.0	0.0	0.0	0.0	0
coffee liqueur	1 oz	118	0.1	0.0	16.1	0.0	0
creme de menthe	1 fl oz	127	0.0	0.0	14.2	0.0	0
daiquiri	2 fl oz	112	0.0	0.0	0.0	0.0	0
gin, 80 proof	1.5 fl oz	97	0.0	0.0	0.0	0.0	0
gin, 90 proof	1.5 fl oz	110	0.0	0	0.0	0.0	0
gin and tonic	7.5 fl oz	171	0.0	0.0	0.0	0.0	0
Irish coffee	6 fl oz	168	5.5	0.0	6.0	0.0	5
mai tai	5.5 fl oz	301	0.0	0.0	29.0	0.0	0
margarita	5.5 fl oz	169	0.0	0.0	10.0	0.0	0
martini	2.5 fl oz	156	0.0	0.0	0.0	0.0	0
piña colada	4.5 fl oz	262	2.7	0.6	40.0		1
rum 80 proof	1.5 fl oz	97	0.0	0.0	0.0	0.0	0
screwdriver	7.5 fl oz	175	0.0	1.1	18.3		0
tequila	1.5 fl oz	97	0.0	0.0	0.0	0.0	0
tequila sunrise	5.5 fl oz	189	0.0	0.5	14.8		0
vodka	1.5 fl oz	97	0.0	0.0	0.0	0.0	0
whiskey	1.5 fl oz	97	0.0	0.0	0.0	0.0	0
wine cooler	5.5 fl oz	100	0.0	0.0	11.4		0
wine, red	3.5 fl oz	74	0.0	0.2	1.8	0.0	0
wine, rosé	3.5 fl oz	73	0.0	0.2	1.4	2.6	0

Food	Portion	Calories	Fat	Protein	Carb	Sugar	Chol
wine spritzer	5.5 fl oz	61	0.0	0.0	1.0		0
wine, white	3.5 fl oz	70	0.0	0.1	0.8	0.6	0

BEVERAGES
CARBONATED BEVERAGES

Food	Portion	Calories	Fat	Protein	Carb	Sugar	Chol
Cherry RC	12 fl oz	160	0.0	0.0	43.0	43.0	0
club soda	12 fl oz	0	0.0	0.0	0.0	0.0	0
Coca-Cola Classic	8 fl oz	97	0.0	0.0	27.0		0
cola	12 fl oz	152	0.0	0.0	38.5		0
cream soda	12 fl oz	189	0.0	0.0	49.3		0
Diet Coke	8 fl oz	1	0.0	0.0	0.0	0.0	0
diet cola	12 fl oz	4	0.0	0.0	0.0	0.0	0
Diet Dr. Pepper	12 fl oz	0	0.0	0.0	0.0	0.0	0
Diet Mountain Dew	12 fl oz	0	0.0	0.0	0.0	0.0	0
Diet Mr. Pibb	8 fl oz	1	0.0	0.0	0.0	0.0	0
Diet Pepsi	12 fl oz	0	0.0	0.0	0.0	0.0	0
Diet RC	12 fl oz	2	0.0	0.0	0.0	0.0	0
Diet Sprite	8 fl oz	3	0.0	0.0	0.0	0.0	0
Dr. Pepper	12 fl oz	150	0.0	0.0	40.0	40.0	0
Fresca	8 fl oz	3	0.0	0.0	0.0	0.0	0
ginger ale	12 fl oz	124	0.0	0.0	31.8		0
grape	12 fl oz	160	0.0	0.0	41.7		0
lemon-lime	12 fl oz	147	0.0	0.0	38.3		0
Mountain Dew	12 fl oz	170	0.0	0.0	46.0	46.0	0
Mr. Pibb	8 fl oz	97	0.0	0.0	26.0		0
orange	12 fl oz	179	0.0	0.0	45.8		0
Pepsi	12 fl oz	150	0.0	0.0	41.0	41.0	0
RC Cola	12 fl oz	160	0.0	0.0	43.2	43.2	0
root beer	12 fl oz	152	0.0	0.0	39.2		0
Seven Up	12 fl oz	144	0.0	0.0	36.2	36.2	0
Sprite	8 fl oz	96	0.0	0.0	26.0		0
Tab	8 fl oz	1	0.0	0.0	0.0	0.0	0

JUICES AND FRUIT-FLAVORED BEVERAGES

Food	Portion	Calories	Fat	Protein	Carb	Sugar	Chol
apple juice	8 fl oz	117	0.0	0.0	29.0	27.0	0
apple/grape juice	8 fl oz	130	0.0	0.0	33.0	31.0	0

Food	Portion	Calories	Fat	Protein	Carb	Sugar	Chol
apple/raspberry juice	8 fl oz	120	0.0	0.0	31.0	28.0	0
apricot nectar	8 fl oz	141	0.0	0.9	36.1		0
Capri Sun juice drink	8 fl oz	122	0.0	0.0	32.2	32.2	0
carrot juice	8 fl oz	99	0.0	2.3	22.8		0
Clamato, Mott's	8 fl oz	110	0.0	1.0	24.0	15.0	0
Cranapple drink, Ocean Spray	8 fl oz	173	0.0	0.0	43.0		0
cranberry juice cocktail	8 fl oz	144	0.0	0.0	36.5		0
crangrape drink, Ocean Spray	8 fl oz	147	0.0	0.0	34.0		0
Crystal Light mix	8 fl oz	5	0.0	0.0	0.0	0.0	0
fruit punch drink	8 fl oz	114	0.0	0.0	28.9		0
grape juice	8 fl oz	154	0.0	1.4	37.8		0
grapefruit juice	8 fl oz	101	0.0	1.4	24.0	25.9	0
Hawaiian Punch	8 fl oz	120	0.0	0.0	30.0	30.0	0
Hawaiian Punch, no sugar added	8 fl oz	15	0.0	0.0	4.0	4.0	0
Kool Aid mix	8 fl oz	100	0.0	0.0	25.0	25.0	0
Kool Aid mix, sugar-free	8 fl oz	5	0.0	0.0	0.0	0.0	0
lemonade, from frozen concentrate	8 fl oz	96	0.0	0.0	25.2	22.1	0
lemonade, from mix	8 fl oz	103	0.0	0.0	26.9	14.5	0
lemonade, from mix, aspartame	8 fl oz	5	0.0	0.0	0.0	0.0	0
lemon juice	1 T	4	0.0	0.0	0.0	0.0	0
lemon juice	8 fl oz	64	0.0	0.9	21.1		0
lime juice	1 T	4	0.0	0.0	1.4	0.0	0
lime juice	8 fl oz	64	0.0	1.1	22.2	5.9	0
orange juice	8 fl oz	112	0.0	1.7	26.8	26.4	0
peach nectar	8 fl oz	134	0.0	0.7	34.7		0
pear nectar	8 fl oz	150	0.0	0.0	39.4		0
pineapple juice	8 fl oz	140	0.0	0.8	34.4	31.3	0

Food	Portion	Calories	Fat	Protein	Carb	Sugar	Chol
prune juice	8 fl oz	182	0.0	1.6	44.7	34.3	0
Sunny Delight Citrus Punch	8 fl oz	125	0.0	0.0	31.5	29.0	0
Tang	8 fl oz	115	0.0	0.0	29.3		0
Tang, sugar-free	8 fl oz	5	0.0	0.0	0.0	0.0	0
tomato juice	8 fl oz	50	0.0	2.0	9.0	7.0	0
V-8 juice cocktail	8 fl oz	50	0.0	1.0	10.0	8.0	0
COFFEE, TEA							
café latte	8 fl oz	117	6.1	6.0	10.0		25
cappucino	8 fl oz	64	3.0	3.0	5.0		14
coffee, brewed	6 fl oz	4	0.0	0.0	1.0		0
coffee, decaffeinated	6 fl oz	4	0.0	0.0	1.0		0
coffee, instant	6 fl oz	4	0.0	0.0	1.0		0
coffee, Cafe Amaretto powder	8 fl oz	60	3.0	8.0	5.0	0.0	0
coffee, Cafe Francais powder	8 fl oz	60	3.5	7.0	5.0	0.0	0
coffee, Cafe Vienna powder	8 fl oz	70	2.5	11.0	10.0	0.0	0
coffee, French Vanilla Cafe powder	8 fl oz	60	2.5	10.0	8.0	0.0	0
coffee, Hazelnut Belgian Cafe powder	8 fl oz	70	2.0	12.0	9.0	0.0	0
coffee, Italian Cappucino powder	8 fl oz	50	1.5	10.0	8.0	0.0	0
coffee, Kahlua Cafe powder	8 fl oz	60	2.0	10.0	7.0	0.0	0
coffee, Swiss Mocha powder	8 fl oz	60	2.5	8.0	6.0	0.0	0
coffee, Viennese Chocolate Cafe powder	8 fl oz	60	2.0	10.0	9.0	0.0	0
tea, black, brewed	6 fl oz	2	0.0	0.0	0.0	0.0	0
tea, green, brewed	6 fl oz	2	0.0	0.0	0.0	0.0	0

Food	Portion	Calories	Fat	Protein	Carb	Sugar	Chol
tea, iced, Nutrasweet, Lipton powder	8 fl oz	5	0.0	0.0	1.0	0.0	0
tea, iced, sugar, lemon, Lipton powder	8 fl oz	90	0.0	0.0	22.0	22.0	0
tea, iced, sweetened, Crystal Light	8 fl oz	70	0.0	0.0	17.0	17.0	0
tea, iced, unsweetened powder	8 fl oz	2	0.0	0.0	0.0	0.0	0

BOX MIXES AND CANNED ENTREES

Food	Portion	Calories	Fat	Protein	Carb	Sugar	Chol
beef and vegetable stew, Armour Star	1 cup	220	12.0	8.0	21.0	0.0	30
beef stew, Hunt	1 cup	155	4.4	14.1	19.6	5.5	21
chicken a la king, Swanson	1 cup	320	22.0	15.0	17.0	2.0	60
chicken teriyaki, LaChoy	1 cup	109	3.0	7.8	15.0	5.2	20
chili with beans, Libby's	1 cup	420	27.0	16.0	29.0	1.0	50
chow mein, beef, LaChoy	1 cup	78	0.8	8.4	10.0	3.0	6
chow mein, chicken, LaChoy	1 cup	80	3.5	7.9	5.7	2.5	9
corned beef hash, Armour Star	1 cup	440	30.0	19.0	23.0	1.0	100
corned beef hash, Libby's	1 cup	470	35.0	21.0	25.0	1.0	90
Hamburger Helper, beef pasta	1 cup	270	10.0	20.0	26.0	2.0	50
Hamburger Helper, beef romanoff	1 cup	290	11.0	20.0	28.0	4.0	50
Hamburger Helper, beef stew	1 cup	250	10.0	18.0	26.0	3.0	50

Food	Portion	Calories	Fat	Protein	Carb	Sugar	Chol
Hamburger Helper, beef taco	1 cup	310	11.0	20.0	30.0	3.0	50
Hamburger Helper, beef teriyaki	1 cup	290	10.0	18.0	34.0	5.0	50
Hamburger Helper, cheddar melt	1 cup	310	12.0	20.0	31.0	4.0	55
Hamburger Helper, cheesy Italian	1 cup	330	14.0	22.0	29.0	6.0	60
Hamburger Helper, cheesy shells	1 cup	340	14.0	22.0	30.0	5.0	60
Hamburger Helper, chili macaroni	1 cup	290	10.0	19.0	30.0	4.0	55
Hamburger Helper, fettucini alfredo	1 cup	310	13.0	20.0	26.0	5.0	55
Hamburger Helper, lasagna	1 cup	280	10.0	19.0	30.0	7.0	50
Hamburger Helper, nacho cheese	1 cup	320	13.0	22.0	30.0	5.0	55
Hamburger Helper, spaghetti	1 cup	300	11.0	21.0	29.0	6.0	55
Hamburger Helper, stroganoff	1 cup	320	13.0	21.0	30.0	7.0	55
Hamburger Helper, Swedish meatball	1 cup	300	14.0	19.0	24.0	2.0	55
Hamburger Helper, zesty Italian	1 cup	320	11.0	21.0	34.0	8.0	55
Hamburger Helper, zesty Mexican	1 cup	300	11.0	19.0	32.0	5.0	50
macaroni and cheese, Kraft	1 cup	390	17.0	11.0	48.0	8.0	10

Food	Portion	Calories	Fat	Protein	Carb	Sugar	Chol
macaroni and cheese, Franco-American	7.5 oz	167	5.4	6.5	23.1		1
noodles, alfredo sauce, Lipton	⅔ cup	250	7.0	10.0	39.0	2.0	75
noodles, butter herb sauce, Lipton	⅔ cup	250	7.0	9.0	41.0	4.0	65
noodles, parmesan sauce, Lipton	⅔ cup	250	8.0	10.0	37.0	2.0	70
noodles, stroganoff sauce, Lipton	⅔ cup	220	4.0	9.0	37.0	2.0	65
Pasta Roni, angel hair, herbs	1 serving	320	3.0	7.0	39.0		0
Pasta Roni, broccoli	1 serving	340	4.0	7.0	37.0		0
Pasta Roni, chicken, broccoli	1 serving	340	4.0	7.0	37.0		0
Pasta Roni, fettucine alfredo	1 serving	460	6.0	9.0	46.0		5
Pasta Roni, four cheese	1 serving	420	6.0	9.0	45.0		5
Pasta Roni, rigatoni, cheddar	1 serving	410	6.0	9.0	46.0		5
Pasta Roni, stroganoff	1 serving	370	7.0	9.0	44.0		5
Pasta and Sauce, alfredo, Lipton	1 serving	330	7.0	40.0	39.0		75
Pasta and Sauce, garlic, Lipton	1 serving	350	6.0	8.0	47.0		10
Pasta and Sauce, cheddar, Lipton	1 serving	320	5.0	9.0	42.0		10
Pasta and Sauce, tomato parmesan, Lipton	1 serving	330	7.0	10.0	39.0		75
pasta salad, caesar, Suddenly Salad	¾ cup	220	9.0	5.0	30.0	4.0	0
pasta salad, classic, Suddenly Salad	¾ cup	220	7.0	5.0	34.0	3.0	0

Food	Portion	Calories	Fat	Protein	Carb	Sugar	Chol
pasta salad, ranch, Suddenly Salad	¾ cup	320	19.0	7.0	31.0	3.0	15
Rice-A-Roni, beef, vermicelli	1 serving	290	1.5	7.0	51.0		0
Rice-A-Roni, broccoli, cheddar	1 serving	370	6.0	8.0	46.0		5
Rice-A-Roni, cheddar, herbs	1 serving	320	5.0	8.0	48.0		5
Rice-A-Roni, chicken, vegetable	1 serving	290	1.0	7.0	51.0		0
Rice-A-Roni, chicken, vermicelli	1 serving	310	1.0	7.0	52.0		0
Rice-A-Roni, chicken, broccoli, vermicelli	1 serving	230	1.0	6.0	40.0		0
Rice-A-Roni, chicken, garlic, vermicelli	1 serving	260	1.0	5.0	42.0		0
Rice-A-Roni, herb, butter	1 serving	320	1.5	6.0	53.0		0
Rice-A-Roni, Mexican-style	1 serving	260	1.5	6.0	40.0		0
Rice-A-Roni, red beans	1 serving	290	1.5	8.0	51.0		0
Rice-A-Roni, rice pilaf	1 serving	310	1.0	7.0	52.0		0
Rice-A-Roni, Spanish rice, vermicelli	1 serving	270	1.0	5.0	41.0		0
rice bowl, beef, broccoli, Uncle Ben's	1 bowl	380	7.0	2.0	58.0		35
rice bowl, sweet/sour chicken, Uncle Ben's	1 bowl	360	3.0	17.0	65.0		30
rice bowl, teriyaki chicken, Uncle Ben's	1 bowl	380	3.5	20.0	66.0		25
rice bowl, teriyaki vegetable, Uncle Ben's	1 bowl	360	3.0	8.0	74.0		0

Food	Portion	Calories	Fat	Protein	Carb	Sugar	Chol
rice, sauce, cheddar, chicken, Lipton	1 serving	280	3.0	7.0	46.0		5
rice, sauce, chicken, Lipton	1 serving	280	2.5	7.0	45.0		5
rice, sauce, mushrooms, Lipton	1 serving	270	1.5	6.0	45.0		0
spaghetti, meat sauce, Kraft	1 cup	330	11.0	12.0	46.0	8.0	15
spaghetti, meat sauce, Franco-American	7.5 oz	211	8.1	8.5	26.2		
Spaghettios, franks	7.5 oz	210	8.4	7.6	26.1		
Spaghettios, meatballs	7.5 oz	202	7.4	9.0	24.8		
Tuna Helper, au gratin	1 cup	310	12.0	14.0	36.0	5.0	20
Tuna Helper, cheesy pasta	1 cup	280	11.0	14.0	32.0	5.0	20
Tuna Helper, creamy broccoli	1 cup	310	12.0	14.0	35.0	6.0	20
Tuna Helper, creamy pasta	1 cup	300	13.0	14.0	31.0	4.0	20
Tuna Helper, fettucine alfredo	1 cup	310	14.0	14.0	32.0	6.0	15
Tuna Helper, tetrazzini	1 cup	310	12.0	17.0	33.0	3.0	20
Tuna Helper, tuna pot pie	1 cup	440	24.0	18.0	40.0	9.0	110
Tuna Helper, tuna romanoff	1 cup	280	8.0	15.0	38.0	3.0	20
BREADS							
bagel	1 bagel	195	1.0	7.5	37.9		0
bagel, cinnamon raisin	1 bagel	155	1.0	6.0	31.0		0

Food	Portion	Calories	Fat	Protein	Carb	Sugar	Chol
bagel, egg	1 bagel	247	1.9	9.0	47.0		21
bagel, whole wheat	1 bagel	150	0.8	6.0	32.0		0
biscuit, plain, refrigerated dough	1 biscuit	49	0.7	1.3	9.7		0
biscuit, buttermilk	1 biscuit	127	5.8	2.2	17.0		0
biscuit, from mix	1 biscuit	191	6.9	4.2	27.6	2.5	2
bread, banana	1 slice	196	6.3	2.6	32.8		26
bread, Boston brown	1 slice	88	0.7	2.3	19.5		9
bread, Bran'ola	1 slice	90	2.0	4.0	18.0	3.0	0
bread, carrot	1 slice	210	10.2	2.9	27.8		24
bread, cinnamon	1 slice	91	2.5	2.2	15.0		0
bread, cracked wheat	1 slice	65	1.0	2.2	12.4		0
bread, French	1 slice	81	1.1	2.7	14.8		
bread, honey wheat berry	1 slice	90	1.5	3.0	19.0	3.0	0
bread, Italian	1 slice	81	1.1	2.6	15.0		0
bread, multigrain	1 slice	65	1.0	2.6	12.1		0
bread, oat bran	1 slice	71	1.3	3.1	11.9		0
bread, potato	1 slice	100	2.0	3.0	18.0	4.0	0
bread, raisin	1 slice	71	1.1	2.1	13.6		0
bread, Roman Meal	1 slice	69	0.9	2.9	13.4		0
bread, rye	1 slice	83	1.1	2.7	15.5		0
bread, sourdough	1 slice	93	0.8	3.7	20.7	1.7	0
bread, wheat	1 slice	90	1.5	4.0	18.0	4.0	0
bread, white	1 slice	67	0.9	2.0	12.4	1.0	0
bread, whole wheat	1 slice	69	1.2	2.7	12.9	1.1	0
bread crumbs	1 cup	427	5.8	13.5	78.3		0
breadsticks, plain	1 stick	41	1.0	1.2	7.0		0
cornbread, from mix	1 slice	18	6.0	4.3	28.9		37
croissant, butter	1 large	272	14.1	5.0	31.0		50
date nut loaf	1 slice	80	2.0	1.0	16.0	5.0	0

Food	Portion	Calories	Fat	Protein	Carb	Sugar	Chol
dinner roll	1 roll	85	2.1	2.4	14.3		0
English muffin, plain	1 muffin	134	1.0	4.4	26.2		0
English muffin, raisin cinnamon	1 muffin	68	0.8	2.0	13.8		0
English muffin, whole wheat	1 muffin	57	0.6	2.0	10.8		0
French toast, frozen	1 piece	126	3.6	4.0	19.0		48
French toast, homemade	1 slice	151	7.3	5.0	16.0		76
hamburger bun	1 bun	123	2.2	3.7	21.6	3.2	0
hotdog roll	1 roll	110	2.0	4.0	21.0		0
kaiser roll	1 roll	167	2.5	5.6	30.0		0
hush puppy	1 piece	74	3.0	1.7	10.1		10
muffin, blueberry	1 muffin	158	3.7	3.1	27.4		17
muffin, blueberry, toaster-type	1 muffin	88	2.7	1.0	14.8		1
muffin, bran	1 muffin	154	4.2	4.0	27.5		0
muffin, corn	1 muffin	174	4.8	3.4	29.0		29
muffin, corn, toaster-type	1 muffin	97	3.2	2.0	15.8		1
muffin, wheat bran, toaster-type	1 muffin	83	2.5	1.0	14.8		3
pancake, blueberry, homemade	1 pancake	84	3.5	2.0	11.0		21
pancake, blueberry, microwave	3 pancakes	230	3.5	5.0	45.0		10
pancake, buckwheat, from mix	1 pancake	62	2.3	2.0	8.0		20
pancake, buttermilk, homemade	1 pancake	86	3.5	3.0	11.0		22
pancake, buttermilk, microwave	3 pancakes	240	4.0	5.0	46.0		10

Food	Portion	Calories	Fat	Protein	Carb	Sugar	Chol
pancake, plain, homemade	1 pancake	86	3.7	2.0	11.0		22
pancake, plain, microwave	3 pancakes	240	1.0	5.0	47.0		10
pita	1 pita	165	0.7	5.5	33.4		0
popover, from mix	1 roll	67	1.5	2.6	10.4		37
pumpernickel	1 slice	80	1.0	2.8	15.3		0
stuffing	½ cup	178	8.6	3.2	21.7		0
Toast-R-Cakes	1 cake	103	3.7	1.7	17.1	8.8	0
tortilla, corn	1 tortilla	56	0.6	1.4	11.7		0
tortilla, flour	1 tortilla	114	2.5	3.0	19.5		0
waffle, apple cinnamon, Eggo	2 waffles	220	7.0	5.0	30.0		20
waffle, Aunt Jemima original	2 waffles	160	4.0	5.0	33.0		0
waffle, blueberry, Eggo	2 waffles	200	7.0	5.0	30.0		20
waffle, blueberry, homemade	1 waffle	186	4.7	6.0	30.0		34
waffle, buttermilk, homemade	1 waffle	217	10.2	6.0	25.0		50
waffle, buttermilk, Eggo	2 waffles	190	7.0	5.0	28.0		20
waffle, buttermilk, Hungry Jack	2 waffles	190	6.0	4.0	29.0		0
waffle, chocolate chip, Eggo	2 waffles	180	6.0	4.0	29.0		20
waffle, cinnamon toast, Eggo	2 waffles	290	10.0	5.0	46.0		25
waffle, homestyle, Hungry Jack	2 waffles	180	6.0	3.0	29.0		0
waffle, Nutri-Grain, Eggo	2 waffles	190	6.0	5.0	30.0		0
BREAKFAST CEREAL							
All-Bran	3.5 oz	81	1.1	3.9	23.0	6.0	0
Alpha-Bits	1 cup	130	1.0	3.0	27.0	13.0	0

Food	Portion	Calories	Fat	Protein	Carb	Sugar	Chol
Apple Jacks	1 cup	120	0.1	1.6	29.6	16.4	0
Banana Nut Crunch	1 cup	250	6.0	5.0	43.0	11.0	0
Basic 4	1 cup	210	3.0	4.0	42.0		0
bran, 100%	½ cup	75	1.4	3.5	20.4		0
Cap'n Crunch	¾ cup	107	1.4	1.4	23.1	11.6	0
Cap'n Crunch, crunchberries	¾ cup	105	1.4	1.2	22.3	12.0	0
Cap'n Crunch, peanut butter	¾ cup	112	2.3	2.0	21.5	9.2	0
Cheerios	1 cup	110	2.0	3.0	23.0	1.0	0
Cheerios, Multi-Grain	1 cup	110	1.0	3.0	24.0	6.0	0
Cocoa Krispies	¾ cup	120	0.8	1.6	27.2	13.0	0
Cocoa Pebbles	¾ cup	120	1.0	1.0	25.0	13.0	0
Cocoa Puffs	1 cup	120	1.0	1.0	27.0	14.0	0
corn flakes, Kellogg's	1 cup	102	0.2	2.3	24.0	1.9	0
corn grits	1 cup	145	0.5	3.4	31.5		0
Corn Pops	1 cup	117	0.2	1.4	27.0	14.0	0
Count Chocula	1 cup	120	1.0	1.0	26.0	14.0	0
cream of rice	¾ cup	95	0.2	1.6	20.9		0
cream of wheat	¾ cup	100	0.4	2.8	20.7		0
crispy rice	1 cup	111	0.1	1.8	24.8	2.5	0
CW Post	¼ cup	122	3.7	2.3	21.0		0
CW Post with raisins	¼ cup	121	4.0	2.4	20.1		0
Dutch Apple	1 cup	220	2.0	4.0	46.0	17.0	0
farina	¾ cup	88	0.2	2.4	18.6	0.2	0
Fiber One	½ cup	60	1.0	2.0	24.0		0
Frankenberry	1 cup	120	1.0	1.0	27.0	14.0	0
Froot Loops	1 cup	120	0.9	1.6	28.2	15.0	0
Frosted Flakes	¾ cup	119	0.2	1.0	28.4	13.0	0
Frosted Mini-Wheats	5 biscuits	180	0.8	4.8	41.0	10.0	0
Fruity Pebbles	¾ cup	110	1.0	1.0	24.0	12.0	0
Golden Crisp	¾ cup	110	0.0	1.0	25.0	15.0	0

Food	Portion	Calories	Fat	Protein	Carb	Sugar	Chol
Golden Grahams	¾ cup	120	1.0	1.0	25.0	11.0	0
granola, Hearty, Post	⅔ cup	280	9.0	5.0	45.0	15.0	0
granola, low-fat, Kellogg's	½ cup	190	2.9	4.1	39.3	12.0	0
granola, Nature Valley	⅓ cup	126	4.9	3.0	18.4		0
granola, oats and honey, Quaker	3.5 oz	219	9.2	5.3	31.4	13.1	1
Grape-Nuts	3.5 oz	200	1.0	6.0	47.0	7.0	0
Heartland Natural	¼ cup	122	4.3	2.8	19.1		0
Honey Bunches of Oats	¾ cup	120	1.5	2.0	25.0	6.0	0
Honey Graham Ohls, Quaker	¾ cup	112	1.9	1.4	22.8	11.1	0
Honey Nut Cheerios	1 cup	120	1.5	3.0	24.0	11.0	0
Honeycomb, Post	1 cup	83	0.0	1.0	19.5	8.3	0
Kix	1 cup	90	0.0	1.0	19.5	2.3	0
Life	¾ cup	121	1.3	3.2	25.2	6.4	0
Lucky Charms	1 cup	120	1.0	2.0	25.0	13.0	0
Maypo	¾ cup	128	1.8	4.3	23.9		0
muesli, 5 grain, Sunbelt	1.9 oz	206	1.9	5.3	41.9	15.3	0
multigrain, Quaker	½ cup	133	1.0	4.5	29.4	0.2	0
Muselix, apple and almond crunch	¾ cup	203	4.8	5.2	39.4	8.9	0
Nutri-Grain, almond raisin	1¼ cups	180	2.8	3.9	38.0	7.0	0
Nutri-Grain, wheat	¾ cup	100	1.0	3.0	24.0		0
oat bran, Common Sense	¾ cup	109	1.2	3.9	23.2	6.3	0
oat bran, cooked	1 cup	198	2.4	7.2	37.8	7.9	0
Oatmeal Crisp, almond	1 cup	220	5.0	6.0	42.0	15.0	0
Oatmeal Crisp, apple	1 cup	210	2.0	4.0	46.0	19.0	0

Food	Portion	Calories	Fat	Protein	Carb	Sugar	Chol
Oatmeal Crisp, raisin	1 cup	210	2.5	4.0	44.0	19.0	0
oatmeal, instant	1 cup	145	2.3	6.1	25.3	0.9	0
oatmeal, instant, apple cinnamon	1 packet	128	1.5	3.3 ·	26.9	10.3	0
oatmeal, instant, cinnamon spice	1 packet	172	2.1	4.1	35.7	15.5	0
oatmeal, instant, raisin spice	1 packet	158	1.9	3.6	32.8	14.7	0
oatmeal, regular/quick	1 cup	145	2.3	6.1	25.3	0.9	0
Product 19	1 cup	100	0.2	2.3	25.1	3.5	0
puffed rice	1 cup	56	0.1	0.9	12.6	0.0	0
puffed wheat	1 cup	51	0.2	2.1	11.1		0
raisin bran, General Mills	¾ cup	200	4.0	4.0	41.0	19.0	0
raisin bran, Kellogg's	1 cup	197	1.5	6.0	47.0	18.0	0
raisin bran, Post	1 cup	190	1.0	4.0	46.0	20.0	0
Rice Krispies	1¼ cups	120	0.2	2.3	28.5	3.0	0
Shredded Wheat, Nabisco	2 biscuits	160	0.5	5.0	38.0	0.0	0
Smacks, Kellogg's	¾ cup	103	0.5	1.7	23.7	14.7	0
Special K	1 cup	110	0.3	6.4	22.4	3.0	0
Sugar Frosted Flakes	¾ cup	109	0.4	1.5	25.2		0
Team Flakes	1¼ cups	220	0.0	4.0	49.0	10.0	0
Total	¾ cup	110	1.0	3.0	24.0	5.0	0
Trix	1 cup	120	1.5	1.0	26.0	13.0	0
Wheatena	¾ cup	102	0.9	3.6	21.5		0
Wheaties	1 cup	110	1.0	3.0	24.0	4.0	0

BURRITOS, TACOS

Food	Portion	Calories	Fat	Protein	Carb	Sugar	Chol
burrito, bacon and egg, Swanson	1 burrito	250	11.0	10.0	27.0	3.0	90
burrito, beans, beef	1 burrito	289	13.0	14.0	30.0		31

Food	Portion	Calories	Fat	Protein	Carb	Sugar	Chol
burrito, beans, beef, Old El Paso	1 burrito	320	10.0	12.0	46.0		15
burrito, beans, beef, Patio	1 burrito	280	7.0	10.0	45.0	5.0	15
burrito, beans, cheese, Old El Paso	1 burrito	290	9.0	12.0	44.0		15
burrito, beans, green chili, Patio	1 burrito	270	7.0	10.0	42.0	3.0	10
burrito, beans, rice	1 burrito	198	3.0	6.0	34.9		3
burrito, beef, cheese, Patio	1 burrito	270	5.0	9.0	46.0	2.0	5
burrito, chicken	1 burrito	286	8.0	24.9	25.9		63
burrito, chicken, Patio	1 burrito	260	4.0	12.0	44.0	5.0	15
burrito, chicken/ cheese, Healthy Choice	1 burrito	360	3.0	16.0	66.0	11.0	15
burrito, ham, cheese, Swanson	1 burrito	210	6.0	9.0	30.0	2.0	100
burrito, hot and spicy, Swanson	1 burrito	220	7.0	9.0	30.0	3.0	55
burrito, sausage, Swanson	1 burrito	240	12.0	9.0	24.0	2.0	90
burrito, scrambled egg, Swanson	1 burrito	200	8.0	8.0	25.0	2.0	60
chiles rellenos	1 serving	426	34.7	23.1	7.0		166
chimichanga, Banquet	1 meal	470	23.0	13.0	56.0		15
chimichanga, beans, cheese	1 chimichanga	258	16.0	8.0	21.1		17
chimichanga, chicken, cheese	1 chimichanga	559	11.0	24.0	31.0		67
chimichanga, chicken, Old El Paso	1 meal	350	16.0	11.0	39.0		20
nachos, cheese	1 oz	64	3.5	2.0	6.1		2

Food	Portion	Calories	Fat	Protein	Carb	Sugar	Chol
nachos, cheese, beans, beef	1 oz	86	4.8	2.0	8.1		12
tamale, meatless	1 tamale	149	8.0	1.0	8.0		6
taco, beef	1 taco	369	20.5	21.0	27.0		56
taco, chicken	1 taco	175	8.3	15.0	10.0		45
taco dinner kit, Old El Paso	1 taco	140	7.0	2.0	19.0		0
taco shell, baked	1 shell	98	4.7	2.0	13.0		0
tortilla, corn	1 tortilla	60	1.0	1.0	12.0		0
tortilla, flour	1 tortilla	150	3.0	4.0	26.0		0
tostada, beef, beans, cheese	1 tostada	168	8.0	8.0	16.1		21
tostada, chicken	1 tostada	125	5.0	8.0	12.9		21
tostada, guacamole	1 tostada	180	12.0	6.0	16.0		20

BUTTER AND SPREADS
BUTTER

Food	Portion	Calories	Fat	Protein	Carb	Sugar	Chol
butter, salted	1 t	36	4.1	0.0	0.0	0.0	11
butter, salted	1 T	108	12.2	0.0	0.0	0.0	33
butter, sweet	1 t	36	4.1	0.0	0.0	0.0	11
butter, sweet	1 T	108	12.2	0.0	0.0	0.0	33
butter, whipped	1 t	29	3.2	0.0	0.0	0.0	9
butter, whipped	1 T	79	8.9	0.0	0.0	0.0	24

MARGARINE

Food	Portion	Calories	Fat	Protein	Carb	Sugar	Chol
Blue Bonnet, 31% oil, soft	1 T	45	5.0	0.0	1.0	0.0	0
Blue Bonnet, 40% oil, stick	1 T	50	6.0	0.0	1.0	0.0	0
Chiffon, 80% oil, soft	1 T	70	7.0	0.0	0.0	0.0	0
Chiffon, 80% oil, whipped	1 T	70	7.0	0.0	0.0	0.0	0
Chiffon Soft	1 T	100	11.0	0.0	0.0	0.0	0
Chiffon, whipped	1 T	70	7.0	0.0	0.0	0.0	0

Food	Portion	Calories	Fat	Protein	Carb	Sugar	Chol
Country Morning Blend, soft	1 T	90	9.0	0.0	0.0	0.0	15
Country Morning Blend, stick	1 T	101	11.3	0.1	0.0	0.0	12
Country Morning Blend, whipped	1 T	94	10.5	0.1	0.0	0.0	11
Fleischmann's, 31% oil, soft	1 T	40	4.5	0.0	1.0	0.0	0
Fleischmann's, 40% oil, stick	1 T	50	6.0	0.0	1.0	0.0	0
Fleischmann's, 80% oil, unsalted, stick	1 T	100	11.0	0.0	0.0	0.0	0
Fleishmann's, stick	1 T	100	11.0	0.0	0.0	0.0	0
Imperial Diet	1 T	49	5.6	0.0	0.0	0.0	0
Imperial Quarters, stick	1 T	107	12.0	0.0	0.1	0.0	0
Imperial soft	1 T	14	11.2	2.3	0.0	0.1	0
Land O' Lakes Corn, stick	1 T	101	11.2	0.0	0.0	0.0	0
Mazola reduced calorie	1 T	50	5.5	0.0	0.0	0.0	0
Mazola stick	1 T	100	11.2	0.0	0.2	0.0	0
Mrs. Filbert's Corn, soft	1 T	100	11.2	0.0	0.1	0.0	0
Mrs. Filbert's Gold	1 T	100	11.2	0.0	0.1	0.0	0
Parkay Diet	1 T	50	6.0	0.0	0.0	0.0	0
Parkay Soft	1 T	100	11.0	0.0	0.0	0.0	0
Parkay, whipped	1 T	70	8.0	0.0	0.0	0.0	0
Shedd's Soft	1 T	99	11.2	0.0	0.0	0.0	0
Shedd's, stick	1 T	78	8.8	0.0	0.0	0.0	0
Shedd's, whipped	1 T	78	8.8	0.0	0.0	0.0	0
MAYONNAISE							
Hellman's	1 T	100	11.0	0.2	0.1	0.0	51
Hellman's light	1 T	50	5.1	0.1	1.0		5
Hellman's reduced calorie	1 T	50	4.9	0.0	1.1		0

Food	Portion	Calories	Fat	Protein	Carb	Sugar	Chol
imitation, soybean	1 T	35	2.9	0.0	2.4		4
Kraft Free	1 T	10	0.0	0.0	2.0	1.0	0
Kraft Light	1 T	50	5.0	0.0	1.0	0.0	0
safflower and soybean	1 T	100	11.1	0.2	0.4		8
soybean	1 T	100	11.1	0.2	0.4		8
SPREADS							
Blue Bonnet, 45% oil, soft	1 T	60	6.0	0.0	0.0	0.0	0
Blue Bonnet, 56% oil, stick	1 T	70	8.0	0.0	0.0	0.0	0
Blue Bonnet, 68% oil	1 T	80	10.0	0.0	0.0	0.0	0
Country Crock, 52% corn oil, soft	1 T	64	7.3	0.0	0.0	0.0	0
Country Crock Classic, 64% oil, stick	1 T	85	9.6	0.0	0.1		0
Country Crock Squeeze	1 T	79	9.0	0.0	0.1		0
Fleischmann's fat-free	1 T	15	0.0	0.0	0.0	0.0	0
Fleischmann's, 56% oil, stick	1 T	70	8.0	0.0	0.0	0.0	0
Fleischmann's 67% oil, soft	1 T	80	9.0	0.0	0.0	0.0	0
Fleischmann's Squeeze, buttery	1 T	5	0.0	0.0	0.0	0.0	0
Imperial Quarters, 60% oil, stick	1 T	79	9.0	0.0	0.1		0
Imperial Savory Squeeze	1 T	86	9.8	0.0	0.1		0
Imperial, whipped	1 T	43	5.0	0.0	0.0	0.0	0
Land O' Lakes, 64% soy oil, soft	1 T	75	9.0	0.0	0.0	0.0	0
Land O' Lakes Sweet Cream Spread	1 T	76	8.4	0.0	0.0	0.0	1

Food	Portion	Calories	Fat	Protein	Carb	Sugar	Chol
Mazola light corn oil	1 T	50	5.6	0.0	0.0	0.0	0
Mrs. Filbert's, 52% corn oil, soft	1 T	64	7.3	0.0	0.0	0.0	0
Mrs. Filbert's 52% oil, soft	1 T	64	7.3	0.0	0.0	0.0	0
Parkay, 40% oil, soft	1 T	50	6.0	0.0	0.0	0.0	0
Parkay, 48% oil, soft	1 T	60	7.0	0.0	0.0	0.0	0
Parkay, 70% oil	1 T	90	10.0	0.0	0.0	0.0	0
Parkay, 70% oil, stick	1 T	90	10.0	0.0	0.0	0.0	0
Parkay Light, 40% oil	1 T	50	6.0	0.0	0.0	0.0	0
Parkay Squeeze, 64% oil	1 T	80	9.0	0.0	0.0	0.0	0
Promise, 53% oil, soft	1 T	65	7.4	0.0	0.0	0.0	0
Promise, 68% oil, soft	1 T	85	9.5	0.0	0.2		0
Promise Extra Lite	1 T	50	5.6	0.2	0.1		0
Promise Quarters, 53% oil, stick	1 T	70	8.0	0.0	0.0	0.0	0
Promise Quarters, 68% oil, stick	1 T	91	10.2	0.0	0.2		0
Shedd's Quarters, 52% oil, stick	1 T	69	7.8	0.0	0.0	0.0	0
Shedd's Spread, 52% oil, soft	1 T	64	7.3	0.0	0.0	0.0	0
CAKES, COOKIES, PIES, PASTRIES							
angel food cake	1 oz	73	0.2	1.7	16.4		0
angel food cake, from mix	1 oz	129	0.1	3.0	29.4		0
animal crackers	1 oz	126	3.9	2.0	21.0	6.4	0
anisette toast	3 cookies	130	1.0	2.0	27.0	17.0	35
apple brown betty	½ cup	230	5.1	2.5	45.5		0

Food	Portion	Calories	Fat	Protein	Carb	Sugar	Chol
apple fritters, frozen	2 fritters	263	12.1	3.3	35.2		
apple pie, frozen	1 slice	296	13.8	2.4	42.5		0
arrowroot biscuit	1 cookie	20	0.0	0.0	3.0	1.0	1
banana cream pie, from mix	1 slice	231	11.9	3.1	29.1		25
banana cream pie, frozen	1 slice	280	14.0	2.0	37.0	25.0	0
blueberry pie, frozen	1 slice	290	12.5	2.3	43.6		0
Boston cream pie, from mix	1 slice	200	4.0	3.0	38.0	28.0	25
Boston cream pie, frozen	1 slice	232	7.8	2.2	39.5		34
Breakfast Treats, Stella D'Oro	1 cookie	100	3.0	1.0	16.0	7.0	10
brown-edge wafers, Nabisco	5 cookies	140	6.0	1.0	21.0	10.0	5
brownie	1 large	227	9.1	2.7	35.8		10
brownie, from mix	2" square	140	6.6	1.4	20.4		9
brownie, from mix, Betty Crocker	1 brownie	180	7.0	2.0	27.0	19.0	20
brownie, from mix, fudge, Duncan Hines	1 brownie	100	2.0	1.0	22.0		0
brownie, fudge, Little Debbie	2.2 oz	269	12.7	2.4	39.2	24.0	13
brownie, fudge, Pillsbury	1.2 oz	139	5.3	1.3	21.6		
butter cookies	1 cookie	23	0.9	0.3	3.4		4
butter pecan cake, from mix	1 slice	250	11.0	3.0	34.0	20.0	55
Cameo cookies, Nabisco	3 cookies	250	9.0	1.0	40.0		0
carrot cake, from mix	1 slice	239	11.0	3.6	32.7		51

Food	Portion	Calories	Fat	Protein	Carb	Sugar	Chol
carrot cake, with cream cheese icing	1 slice	484	29.3	5.1	52.4		60
cheesecake	1 slice	257	18.0	4.4	20.4		44
cheesecake, mix, no-bake	1 slice	271	12.6	5.4	35.1		42
cherry pie, frozen	1 slice	325	13.8	2.5	49.8		0
chocolate cake, from mix	1 slice	198	7.6	3.6	31.9		35
chocolate chip cookies	1 cookie	78	3.5	0.9	9.3		0
chocolate chip cookies, chewy	3 cookies	170	8.0	1.0	23.0	14.0	5
chocolate chip cookies, Chips Deluxe, Keebler	1 cookie	80	4.5	1.0	9.0		0
chocolate chip cookies, from mix	1 cookie	79	4.1	0.9	10.3		7
chocolate chip cookies, from dough	1 cookie	59	2.7	0.6	8.2		3
chocolate chip cookies, Soft Batch, Keebler	1 cookie	80	3.5	1.0	10.0		0
chocolate cream pie, frozen	1 slice	344	21.9	2.9	38.0		6
chocolate fudge sandwich	1 cookie	83	3.7	0.9	11.7		0
chocolate pudding cake, from mix	1 slice	270	14.3	3.5	34.2		53
chocolate sandwich cookie	1 cookie	47	2.1	0.5	7.0		0
chocolate snack cake with creme	1 cake	188	7.3	1.7	30.1		9
chocolate wafers, Nabisco	1 oz	140	4.0	1.9	20.5	11.5	5
coconut cream pie, frozen	1 slice	191	10.6	9.0			0
coffee cake, cinnamon, from mix	1 slice	178	5.4	3.1	29.6		27

Food	Portion	Calories	Fat	Protein	Carb	Sugar	Chol
coffee cake, snack	1 cake	227	7.2				8
croissant	1 medium	231	12.0	4.7	26.1		43
cruller, glazed	1 cruller	169	7.5	1.3	24.4		5
cupcake, chocolate with icing	1 cupcake	173	6.5	2.0	27.9		
cupcake, chocolate, creme-filled	1 cupcake	185	9.4	1.7	25.9	17.6	4
danish pastry, cheese	1 pastry	266	15.5	5.7	26.4		32
danish pastry, fruit	1 pastry	263	13.1	3.8	33.9		15
devil's food cake, from mix	1 slice	190	5.0	2.0	33.0		0
doughnut, cake	1 doughnut	198	10.8	2.3	23.4	7.9	17
doughnut, cake, glazed	1 doughnut	192	10.3	2.3	22.9		14
doughnut, yeast, jelly	1 doughnut	289	15.9	5.0	33.1		22
eclair, chocolate	1 eclair	196	9.2	2.6	25.5		25
E.L. Fudge cookies, Keebler	2 cookies	120	5.0	1.0	17.0		0
fig newton	2 cookies	110	2.5	1.0	20.0	13.0	0
fruitcake	1 slice	139	3.9	1.2	26.5	18.5	2
fudge cake, from mix	1 slice	320	17.0	3.0	40.0	28.0	80
fudge sticks, Keebler	3 cookies	150	8.0	1.0	19.0		0
gingerbread, from mix	1 slice	207	6.8	2.7	34.0		23
gingersnaps	4 cookies	118	2.8	1.6	21.8		0
gingersnaps, Keebler	5 cookies	150	6.0	2.0	24.0		0
golden cake, from mix	1 slice	320	16.0	3.0	42.0	29.0	80
graham crackers, chocolate-coated	1 oz	137	6.6	1.6	18.9		0
graham crackers, chocolate snack	25 pieces	140	5.0	2.0	23.0	8.0	0

Food	Portion	Calories	Fat	Protein	Carb	Sugar	Chol
graham crackers, cinnamon	5 crackers	140	3.0	2.0	26.0	11.0	0
graham crackers, fudge, Keebler	3 crackers	140	7.0	1.0	19.0		0
graham crackers, honey	4 crackers	120	2.9	2.0	21.8		0
Grasshopper mint fudge cookies, Keebler	4 cookies	150	7.0	2.0	19.0		0
key lime pie, frozen	1 slice	380	14.0	5.0	58.0	45.0	15
lemon chiffon, from mix	1 slice	140	3.0	3.0	26.0	16.0	25
lemon meringue pie, frozen	1 slice	303	9.8	1.7	53.3		51
lemon pudding cake, from mix	1 slice	180	4.0	2.0	33.0	24.0	35
Lorna Doone cookies, Nabisco	4 cookies	140	7.0	2.0	19.0	6.0	5
Mallomars, Nabisco	2 cookies	120	5.0	1.0	17.0	13.0	0
marble cake, from mix	1 slice	253	12.4	3.1	34.5		53
molasses cookies	1 cookie	65	1.9	0.8	11.1		0
Mystic Mint cookies, Nabisco	1 cookie	90	4.0	1.0	11.0	8.0	0
Nilla Wafers, Nabisco	8 cookies	140	5.0	2.0	24.0	12.0	0
Nutter Butter, Nabisco	2 cookies	130	6.0	2.0	19.0	8.0	5
oatmeal cookies	1 cookie	81	3.3	1.1	12.4		0
oatmeal cookies, from mix	1 cookie	74	3.1	1.2	10.4		7
oatmeal cookies, from dough	1 cookie	57	2.5	0.7	7.9		3
oatmeal cookies, soft	1 cookie	61	2.2	0.9	9.9		1
oatmeal raisin cookies	1 cookie	65	2.4	1.0	10.3		5

Food	Portion	Calories	Fat	Protein	Carb	Sugar	Chol
oatmeal raisin cookies, from mix	2 cookies	130	6.0	2.0	18.0	0	
Oreo cookies, Nabisco	2 cookies	160	7.0	2.0	23.0	13.0	
peach pie, frozen	1 slice	261	11.7	2.2	38.5		0
peanut butter cookies	1 cookie	72	3.5	1.4	8.8		0
peanut butter cookies, from dough	1 cookie	60	3.3	1.1	6.9		4
peanut butter cookies, from mix	2 cookies	140	7.3	1.8	11.8		0
pecan pie	1 slice	452	20.9	4.5	64.6		36
Pecan Shortbread Sandies, Keebler	1 cookie	80	5.0	1.0	9.0		1
pineapple upside-down, from mix	1 slice	400	15.0	3.0	63.0	43.0	35
pound cake, butter	1 slice	116	6.0	1.6	14.6		66
pound cake, frozen	1 slice	131	7.0	1.5	15.5		
pumpkin pie, frozen	1 slice	229	10.4	4.3	29.8		22
shortbread cookies	1 cookie	40	1.9	0.5	1.1		2
shortbread pecan cookies	1 cookie	76	4.6	0.7	8.2		5
spice, from mix	1 slice	250	11.0	3.0	35.0	20.0	55
sponge cake	1 slice	187	2.7	2.1	23.2		107
strudel	1 slice	195	8.0	2.3	29.2		20
sugar cookies	1 cookie	72	3.2	0.8	10.2		8
sugar cookies, from dough	1 cookie	58	2.8	0.6	7.9		4
sugar cookies, from mix	2 cookies	130	6.0	1.2	16.8		0
sugar wafers, chocolate filling, Keebler	3 wafers	140	7.0	1.0	18.0		0
sugar wafers, creme filling	8 wafers	145	6.9	1.2	19.9		0

Food	Portion	Calories	Fat	Protein	Carb	Sugar	Chol
sugar wafers, creme filling, Keebler	3 wafers	130	6.0	1.0	19.0		0
sweet potato pie, frozen	1 slice	280	11.0	4.0	43.0	22.0	40
toaster pastry, apple cinnamon, Pop Tarts	1 pastry	200	5.0	2.3	37.0	15.0	0
toaster pastry, blueberry, Pop Tarts	1 pastry	200	5.0	2.0	36.0	14.0	0
toaster pastry, cherry, Pop Tarts	1 pastry	204	5.0	2.0	37.0	15.0	0
turnover, apple	1 turnover	170	7.9	2.0	22.8		
turnover, blueberry	1 turnover	166	7.9	2.0	21.4		
turnover, cherry	1 turnover	173	7.9	2.1	23.2		
vanilla sandwich with creme filling	1 cookie	48	2.0	0.5	7.2		0
vanilla wafers	4 cookies	74	3.3	0.8	10.1		0
Vienna Fingers	2 cookies	140	6.0	2.0	21.0		0
white cake, from mix	1 slice	190	4.8	2.5	34.3		0
white pudding cake, from mix	1 slice	244	10.2	2.5	35.7		0
yellow cake, from mix	1 slice	202	5.9	3.0	34.3		37
yellow pudding cake, from mix	1 slice	243	11.0	3.1	33.2		50
CANDY							
After Eight Mints	2 mints	29	1.1	0.0	6.1		0
Almond Joy	1.7 oz bar	241	13.1	2.1	28.6	22.3	2
Baby Ruth	2.1 oz bar	289	12.7	4.5	39.1		2
Bar None	1.5 oz bar	224	14.6	3.5	22.4		7
Bit-O-Honey	2.1 oz bar	186	3.8	1.4	38.9	23.1	0
Butterfinger	2.2 oz bar	293	11.4	7.6	40.0		1
candy corn	¼ cup	182	1.0	0.0	44.8		0

Food	Portion	Calories	Fat	Protein	Carb	Sugar	Chol
caramels	2.5 oz	272	5.8	3.3	54.7		5
chocolate, milk	1.55 oz bar	226	13.5	11.9	178.0	91.0	10
chocolate, semi-sweet (baking)	1 oz	228	14.3	2.0	30.1	15.3	0
chocolate, sweet	1.45 oz bar	207	14.0	1.6	24.4	20.0	0
chocolate chips, semi-sweet	1 cup	1351	84.7	11.9	178.1	90.7	0
Chunky	1.4 oz bar	198	11.7	3.6	22.8		4
Crunch	1.4 oz bar	209	10.5	2.4	26.1		5
Fifth Avenue	2 oz bar	197	8.5	3.6	26.4	18.0	2
fudge, chocolate	6 oz piece	65	1.4	0.0	13.0		2
Goobers	1.38 oz	200	13.1	5.3	5.7	2.0	4
Gummi Bears	1.39 oz	129	0.0	2.2	30.0	18.6	0
Hershey milk chocolate	1.5 oz bar	233	13.4	3.2	24.9	21.7	9
jelly beans	10 large	103	0.1	0.0	26.1	16.5	0
Kisses, Hershey	8 pieces	211	7.7	2.9	22.6	19.7	8
Kit Kat Wafer	1.5 oz bar	219	11.2	2.9	26.7	22.4	8
Krackel	1.5 oz bar	218	11.8	2.7	25.3	20.7	8
M&Ms	1.69 oz pkg	236	10.1	2.1	34.2		7
M&Ms Peanut	1.7 oz pkg	253	12.9	4.6	29.6		4
Mars Almond	1.76 oz bar	234	11.5	4.0	31.4		5
marshmallows	1 regular	23	0.0	0.0	5.9		0
Milky Way	2.15 oz bar	258	9.8	2.7	43.7		9
Mounds	1.9 oz bar	253	13.3	2.0	31.2	20.9	1
Mr. Goodbar	1.75 oz bar	252	15.8	6.2	25.1		10
Oh Henry	2 oz bar	244	9.6	6.2	36.7		5
peanut brittle	1 oz	128	5.4	2.1	19.6		4
Peanut Butter Cups, Reese's	2 pieces	270	15.6	5.2	27.3	23.6	3
Peppermint Pattie, York	1.5 oz patty	165	3.0	1.0	33.6	26.6	0
Planters Peanut Bar	1.6 oz bar	230	14.0	6.0	22.0	13.0	0
Raisinets	1.58 oz	185	7.2	2.1	32.0		2
Reese's Pieces	1.6 oz pkg	226	9.7	6.4	28.2	24.3	1

Food	Portion	Calories	Fat	Protein	Carb	Sugar	Chol
Rolo caramels	9 pieces	219	10.6	2.6	28.4	25.5	9
Skittles	2.3 oz	263	2.8	0.0	58.9		0
Skor toffee bar	1.4 oz bar	219	13.4	1.8	22.7	21.0	20
Snickers	2.16 oz bar	292	15.0	4.9	36.1		8
Starburst Fruit Chews	6 pieces	234	4.9	0.2	49.9		0
Symphony	1.4 oz bar	209	13.0	3.1	22.7		11
Three Musketeers	2.13 oz bar	250	7.7	1.9	46.1		7
Twix, caramel	2 oz pkg	283	13.8	2.6	37.2		3
Twizzlers, Cherry Twists	1.43 oz	136	0.8	1.3	31.0	16.5	0
Twizzlers, Strawberry	2.5 oz pkg	263	1.1	2.3	65.8		0

CHEESE AND CHEESE PRODUCTS

Food	Portion	Calories	Fat	Protein	Carb	Sugar	Chol
American cheese, processed	1 oz	106	8.9	6.3	0.5		27
American cheese, processed, Kraft	1 oz slice	110	9.0	5.0	1.0		25
American cheese food	1 oz	93	7.0	5.6	2.1	2.8	18
American cheese food, Kraft	¾ oz slice	70	5.0	4.0	2.0	1.0	15
blue	1 oz	100	8.1	6.1	0.7		21
brick	1 oz	105	8.4	6.6	0.8		27
Brie	1 oz	95	7.8	5.9	0.1		28
Camembert	1 oz	85	6.9	5.6	0.1		20
cheddar	1 oz	114	9.4	7.1	0.1		30
cheddar, shredded	1 cup	455	37.4	28.1	1.4		119
cheddar, low-fat	1 oz	49	2.0	6.9	0.5		6
cheddar, low-sodium	1 oz	113	9.2	6.9	0.5		28
cheese sauce, cheddar, Land O'Lakes	1 oz	38	2.5	0.7	2.5		5
cheese spread, American	1 oz	82	6.0	4.7	2.5		16

Food	Portion	Calories	Fat	Protein	Carb	Sugar	Chol
cheese spread, Cheez Whiz	2 T	90	7.0	5.0	2.0	2.0	20
cheese spread, Velveeta	1 oz	80	6.0	5.0	3.0	2.0	20
Cheshire	1 oz	110	8.7	6.6	1.4		29
Colby	1 oz	112	9.1	6.7	0.7		27
cottage cheese, 1% fat	1 cup	164	2.3	28.0	6.1		10
cottage cheese, 2% fat	1 cup	203	4.4	31.1	8.2		19
cottage cheese, creamed	1 cup	217	9.5	26.2	5.6		31
cottage cheese, dry curd	1 cup	123	0.6	25.0	2.7		10
cream cheese	1 oz	99	9.9	2.1	0.8		31
cream cheese, fat-free	1 oz	30	0.0	5.0	2.0	1.0	5
cream cheese, whipped	3 T	110	11.0	2.0	1.0	1.0	35
Edam	1 oz	101	7.9	7.1	0.4		25
farmers	1 oz	100	8.0	6.0	1.0		25
feta	1 oz	75	6.0	4.0	1.2		25
fontina	1 oz	110	8.8	7.3	0.4		33
goat, soft	1 oz	76	6.0	4.1	1.4		13
Gouda	1 oz	101	7.8	5.0	2.2		32
Gruyère	1 oz	117	9.2	8.5	0.1		31
Havarti	1 oz	120	11.0	6.0	0.0		35
jalapeno jack, processed	1 oz	90	8.0	5.0	1.0		20
Monterey jack, processed	1 oz	106	8.6	6.9	0.2		25
mozzarella, part skim	1 oz	72	4.5	6.9	0.8		16
mozzarella, string	1 oz stick	80	6.0	7.0	1.0		20
mozzarella, whole milk	1 oz	80	6.1	5.5	0.6		22
Muenster	1 oz	104	8.5	6.6	0.3		27
Neufchâtel	1 oz	74	6.6	2.8	0.8		22

Food	Portion	Calories	Fat	Protein	Carb	Sugar	Chol
parmesan, grated	1 T	23	1.5	2.1	0.2		4
provolone	1 oz	100	7.5	7.3	0.6		20
ricotta, part skim	½ cup	171	9.8	14.1	6.4	1.7	38
ricotta, whole milk	½ cup	216	16.1	14.0	3.8	1.7	63
Romano, grated	1 oz	110	7.6	9.0	1.0		29
Roquefort, sheep's milk	1 oz	105	8.7	6.1	0.6		26
Swiss	1 oz	107	7.8	8.1	1.0		26
Swiss, Kraft	1 slice	70	5.0	4.0	1.0	1.0	15
Swiss cheese food	1 oz	92	6.8	6.2	1.3		23
Swiss, processed	1 oz	95	7.1	7.0	0.6		24
CONDIMENTS							
A1 Steak Sauce	1 T	15	0.0	0.0	3.0	2.0	0
barbeque sauce	1 T	12	0.0	0.0	2.0		0
chili sauce	1 T	18	0.0	1.0	8.0		0
horseradish, prepared	1 T	6	0.0	0.0	1.4		0
hot sauce	1 t	1	0.0	0.0	0.0	0.0	0
ketchup	1 T	16	0.0	0.0	4.0	3.5	0
mayonnaise	1 T	100	11.0	0.0	0.0		51
mustard	1 t	5	0.0	0.0	0.0	0.0	0
pepper sauce, Tabasco	1 t	1	0.0	0.0	0.0	0.0	0
pickle relish	1 T	20	0.0	0.0	6.0	6.0	0
pickles, bread and butter	4 slices	19	0.0	0.0	4.3	3.3	0
pickles, dill	4 slices	5	0.0	0.0	0.0	0.0	0
pickles, sweet	4 slices	40	0.0	0.0	10.0	10.0	0
salsa, mild	2 T	30	0.0	0.0	6.0	1.5	0
soy sauce	1 T	11	0.0	1.5	1.0	1.0	0
steak sauce	1 T	10	0.0	0.0	2.3	1.5	0
sweet and sour sauce, Kikkoman	1 T	17	0.0	0.0	4.3		0
tamari sauce	1 T	11	0.0	2.0	1.0		0
tartar sauce	2 T	100	10.0	0.0	4.0		50

Food	Portion	Calories	Fat	Protein	Carb	Sugar	Chol
teriyaki sauce	1 T	15	0.0	0.0	3.2		0
Worcestershire sauce	1 t	5	0.0	0.0	1.0	1.0	0

CRACKERS

Food	Portion	Calories	Fat	Protein	Carb	Sugar	Chol
Better Cheddars	22 crackers	150	7.0		18.0		5
Big Town	10 crackers	237	7.9	2.7	38.6		
Cheese Nips	32 crackers	130	4.0	3.0	21.0		5
Cheez-It	15 crackers	160	8.0	4.0	16.0		0
Chicken in a Biskit	12 crackers	160	9.0		17.0		0
Club	4 crackers	70	3.0	1.0	9.0	1.0	0
Crown Pilot	1 cracker	70	1.5	1.0	13.0		0
Garden Crisps	15 crackers	130	3.5	2.0	22.0		0
Harvest Crisps	13 crackers	130	3.5	3.0	23.0		0
Hi Ho Crackers	4 crackers	70	4.0	1.0	8.0	1.0	0
Melba toast	1 round	12	0.1	0.0	2.0		0
milk	1 cracker	55	1.9	0.9	8.4		2
Oat Thins	18 crackers	140	6.0	3.0	20.0		0
oyster	23 crackers	60	1.5	1.0	11.0		0
Ritz	5 crackers	80	4.0	1.0	10.0		0
Ritz Bitz sandwiches, cheese	14 crackers	160	10.0	3.0	17.0		5
Ritz Bitz sandwiches, peanut butter	13 crackers	150	8.0	4.0	17.0		0
Royal Lunch	15 crackers	50	2.0	1.0	8.0		0
rye crispbread	1 cracker	37	0.1	0.8	8.2		0
saltines	5 crackers	60	1.5	1.0	10.0		0
Snackwell's, cheese	15 crackers	60	1.0	1.5	11.0		5
Snackwell's, wheat	15 crackers	70	1.5	2.0	11.0		0
Sociables	7 crackers	80	4.0	1.0	9.0		0
Town House Crackers	5 crackers	80	4.5	1.0	9.0	1.0	0
Triscuit wafers	7 crackers	140	5.0	3.0	21.0		0

Food	Portion	Calories	Fat	Protein	Carb	Sugar	Chol
Uneeda	2 crackers	60	1.5	1.0	11.0		0
Vegetable Thins	14 crackers	160	9.0	2.0	19.0		0
Wasa Crisp	2 crackers	50	0.0	2.0	10.0		0
Waverly	5 crackers	70	3.5	1.0	10.0		0
Wheatables	16 crackers	140	6.0	2.0	20.0	4.0	0
Wheat Thins	18 crackers	120	4.0	2.0	21.0		0
Zesta	2 crackers	26	0.7	0.6	4.3		0
zwieback	1 cracker	35	1.0	1.0	6.0	1.0	0

CREAMS AND CREAM SUBSTITUTES

Food	Portion	Calories	Fat	Protein	Carb	Sugar	Chol
cream, light	1 T	29	2.9	0.4	0.5		10
cream, whipping, heavy	1 T	52	5.5	0.3	0.4	0.4	21
cream, whipping, light	1 T	44	4.6	0.3	0.4		17
cream, whipping, pressurized	1 T	8	0.7	0.1	0.4		2
creamer, liquid, Coffee-Mate	1 T	20	1.0	0.0	2.0	0.0	0
creamer, liquid, Coffee Rich	½ oz	22	1.6	0.0	2.2		0
creamer, powdered	1 t	11	0.7	0.1	1.1		0
creamer, powdered, Coffee-Mate	1 t	10	0.6	0.0	2.0	0.0	0
half and half	1 T	20	1.7	0.4	0.6		6
sour cream, cultured	1 T	26	2.5	0.4	0.5		5
sour cream, fat-free	2 T	35	0.0		6.0	2.0	20
sour cream, light	2 T	40	2.5	2.0	2.0	2.0	10
sour cream dip, Breakstone	2 T	54	4.2	1.0	2.0	1.0	21
sour cream dip, Kraft	2 T	60	4.1	1.0	3.4	0.0	0

Food	Portion	Calories	Fat	Protein	Carb	Sugar	Chol
sour cream dip, French onion, Sealtest	2 T	50	4.0	1.0	2.0	1.0	20
whipped topping, frozen	1 T	13	1.0	0.1	0.9		0
whipped topping, frozen, Cool Whip	2 T	25	1.5	0.0	2.0	2.0	0
whipped topping, Kraft	2 T	20	1.5	0.0	1.0	1.0	0
whipped topping, pressurized	1 T	11	0.9	0.0	0.6		0

FAST FOODS

ARBY'S

Food	Portion	Calories	Fat	Protein	Carb	Sugar	Chol
biscuit, bacon	1 sandwich	360	24	9	27		10
biscuit, butter	1 sandwich	280	17	5	27		0
biscuit, ham	1 sandwich	330	20	12	28		30
biscuit, sausage	1 sandwich	460	33	12	28		25
chicken fingers	medium	580	32	19	55		35
chicken sandwich, bacon, Swiss	1 sandwich	610	33	31	49		110
chicken sandwich, breast fillet	1 sandwich	540	30	24	47		90
chicken sandwich, cordon bleu	1 sandwich	630	35	34	47		120
chicken sandwich, grilled deluxe	1 sandwich	450	22	29	37		110
chicken sandwich, roast club	1 sandwich	340	13	29	38		90
croissant, ham	1 sandwich	310	19	13	29		50
croissant, sausage	1 sandwich	440	32	13	29		45
croissant, bacon	1 sandwich	340	23	10	28		30
french fries, cheddar curly	medium	460	24	6	54		5
french fries, curly	small	310	15	4	39		0
french fries, curly	medium	400	20	5	40		0
french fries, curly	large	620	30	8	78		0

Food	Portion	Calories	Fat	Protein	Carb	Sugar	Chol
french fries, homestyle	small	300	13	3	42		0
french fries, homestyle	medium	370	16	4	53		0
french fries, homestyle	large	560	24	6	79		0
grilled chicken, light	7.5 oz	280	5	29	30		55
ham and Swiss sandwich, hot	1 sandwich	340	13	23	35		90
jalapeno bites	medium	330	21	7	30		40
market sandwich, roast beef, Swiss	1 sandwich	810	42	37	73		130
market sandwich, ham, Swiss	1 sandwich	730	34	36	74		125
market sandwich, chicken caesar	1 sandwich	820	38	43	75		140
market sandwich, turkey, Swiss	1 sandwich	760	33	43	75		130
mozzarella sticks	5 oz	470	29	18	34		60
onion petals	4 oz	410	24	4	43		0
potato, broccoli, cheddar	1 potato	540	24	12	71		50
potato cakes	2 cakes	250	16	2	26		4
roast chicken deluxe, light	7.2 oz	260	5	23	33		40
roast beef sandwich, Arby's Melt	1 sandwich	340	15	16	36		70
roast beef sandwich, Arby-Q	1 sandwich	360	14	16	40		70
roast beef sandwich, beef, cheddar	1 sandwich	480	24	23	43		90
roast beef sandwich, Big Montana	1 sandwich	630	32	47	41		155
roast beef sandwich, giant	1 sandwich	480	23	32	41		110

Food	Portion	Calories	Fat	Protein	Carb	Sugar	Chol
roast beef sandwich, junior	1 sandwich	310	13	16	34		70
roast beef sandwich, regular	1 sandwich	350	16	21	34		85
roast beef sandwich, super	1 sandwich	470	23	22	47		85
roast turkey deluxe, light	7.2 oz	260	5	23	33		40
salad, caesar	1 salad	90	4	7	8		10
salad, chicken caesar	1 salad	230	8	33	8		80
salad, chicken finger	1 salad	570	34	30	39		65
salad, garden	1 salad	70	1	4	14		0
salad, grilled chicken	1 salad	210	5	30	14		65
salad, roast chicken	1 salad	160	3	20	15		40
salad, turkey club	1 salad	350	21	33	9		90
shake, chocolate	medium	480	16	10	84		45
shake, jamocha	medium	470	15	10	82		45
shake, strawberry	medium	500	13	11	87		15
shake, vanilla	medium	470	15	10	83		45
sourdough, bacon	1 sandwich	420	10	16	66		10
sourdough, ham	1 sandwich	390	6	19	67		30
sourdough, sausage	1 sandwich	520	19	19	67		25
sub sandwich, French dip	1 sandwich	440	18	28	42		100
sub sandwich, hot ham, Swiss	1 sandwich	530	27	29	45		110
sub sandwich, Italian	1 sandwich	780	53	29	49		120
sub sandwich, Philly beef, Swiss	1 sandwich	700	42	36	46		130
sub sandwich, roast beef	1 sandwich	760	48	35	47		130
sub sandwich, turkey	1 sandwich	630	37	26	51		100

Food	Portion	Calories	Fat	Protein	Carb	Sugar	Chol
turnover, apple	1 turnover	420	16	4	65		0
turnover, cherry	1 turnover	410	16	4	63		0
BOSTON MARKET							
apples, hot cinnamon	¾ cup	250	5	0	56	49	0
baked beans, BBQ	¾ cup	270	5	8	48	20	0
black beans and rice	1 cup	300	10	8	45	3	0
broccoli rice casserole	¾ cup	240	12	5	26	2	40
brownie, chocolate	1 brownie	310	10	3	51	26	5
butternut squash	¾ cup	150	6	2	25	12	20
cake, chocolate	1 slice	510	24	3	73	63	25
cake, hummingbird	1 slice	710	36	6	92	75	85
carrots, glazed	¾ cup	280	15	1	35	9	0
cheesecake	1 slice	580	41	9	44	32	165
chicken, ¼ dark, skinless	¼ chicken	190	10	22	1	1	115
chicken, ¼ dark, with skin	¼ chicken	320	21	22	1	1	155
chicken, ¼ white, skinless	¼ chicken	170	4	33	2	1	85
chicken, ¼ white, with skin	¼ chicken	280	12	33	2	1	135
chicken caesar salad	1 salad	810	60	43	25	4	105
chicken pot pie	1 pie	750	46	26	57	4	110
chicken salad, chunky	1 salad	480	39	25	4	3	110
chicken salad sandwich	1 sandwich	680	30	39	63	12	120
chicken sandwich	1 sandwich	390	5	31	60	12	55
chicken sandwich, BBQ	1 sandwich	540	9	30	84	33	75

Food	Portion	Calories	Fat	Protein	Carb	Sugar	Chol
chicken sandwich, cheese, sauce	1 sandwich	630	28	37	61	13	90
cole slaw	¾ cup	300	19	2	30	26	20
cookie, chocolate chip	1 cookie	390	19	3	33	13	15
cookie, oatmeal	1 cookie	390	20	5	47	24	30
cookie, peanut butter	1 cookie	420	25	7	43	26	20
corn, herb buttered	¾ cup	180	4	5	30	12	0
corn, whole kernel	¾ cup	180	4	5	30	13	0
cornbread	1 loaf	200	6	3	33	13	25
cranberry relish	¾ cup	350	5	1	15	14	0
cranberry walnut relish	¾ cup	350	5	3	75	66	0
cucumber salad	¾ cup	120	10	2	9	2	0
fruit salad	¾ cup	70	1	1	15	14	0
green beans	¾ cup	60	6	1	5	2	0
green beans, casserole	¾ cup	80	4.5	1	9	3	5
ham, honey glazed	5 oz	210	8	24	10	10	75
ham sandwich	1 sandwich	410	8	25	65	5	45
ham sandwich, cheese, sauce	1 sandwich	650	31	31	67	18	85
macaroni and cheese	¾ cup	280	11	13	33	8	30
meatloaf	5 oz	290	17	20	15	4	70
meatloaf sandwich, cheese	1 sandwich	690	27	36	83	18	90
meatloaf sandwich, open-faced	1 meal	730	36	29	74	7	95
pie, apple streusel	1 slice	480	18	4	63	30	15
pie, cherry streusel	1 slice	410	17	4	60	21	10

Food	Portion	Calories	Fat	Protein	Carb	Sugar	Chol
pie, pecan	1 slice	550	27	5	71	36	110
pie, pumpkin	1 slice	370	17	5	50	35	50
potatoes, garlic and dill	¾ cup	130	2.5	3	25	2	0
potatoes, mashed	¾ cup	210	9	4	32	4	25
potatoes, new	¾ cup	130	3	3	25	2	0
potato salad	¾ cup	200	12	3	22	5	15
red beans and rice	1 cup	260	5	8	45	2	5
rice pilaf	⅔ cup	180	5	5	32	0	0
side salad, Caesar	4 oz	200	17	7	7	2	15
spinach, creamed	¾ cup	260	20	9	11	2	55
squash casserole	¾ cup	330	24	7	20	8	70
stuffing, savory	¾ cup	310	12	6	44	3	0
sweet potato casserole	¾ cup	280	18	3	39	23	10
tortellini salad	¾ cup	350	24	11	24	3	55
turkey bacon club sandwich	1 sandwich	780	38	47	64	15	145
turkey breast, skinless	5 oz	170	1	36	1	0	100
turkey sandwich	1 sandwich	390	3.5	33	61	13	60
turkey sandwich, cheese, sauce	1 sandwich	620	25	39	64	14	110
turkey sandwich, open-faced	1 meal	720	20	47	64	15	105
vegetables, steamed	⅔ cup	35	1	2	7	3	0
BURGER KING							
biscuit with bacon, egg, cheese	1 biscuit	510	31.0	19.0	39.0	3.0	225
biscuit with sausage	1 biscuit	590	40.0	16.0	41.0	2.0	45
cheeseburger	1 sandwich	380	19.0	23.0	28.0	5.0	65
cheeseburger, double	1 sandwich	600	36.0	41.0	28.0	5.0	135

Food	Portion	Calories	Fat	Protein	Carb	Sugar	Chol
cheeseburger, double with bacon	1 sandwich	640	39.0	44.0	28.0	5.0	145
chicken sandwich	1 sandwich	710	43.0	26.0	54.0	4.0	60
Chicken Tenders	8 pieces	310	17.0	21.0	19.0	3.0	50
Croissandwich, sausage, egg, cheese	1 sandwich	600	46.0	22.0	25.0	3.0	260
fish sandwich	1 sandwich	700	41.0	26.0	56.0	4.0	90
french fries	medium	370	20.0	5.0	43.0	0.0	0
french toast sticks	1 serving	500	27.0	4.0	60.0	11.0	0
hamburger	1 sandwich	330	15.0	20.0	28.0	4.0	55
hash browns	1 serving	220	12.0	2.0	25.0	0.0	0
onion rings	1 serving	310	14.0	4.0	41.0	6.0	0
pie, apple	1 serving	300	15.0	3.0	39.0	22.0	0
salad, chicken	1 serving	200	10.0	21.0	7.0	4.0	60
salad, garden	1 serving	100	5.0	6.0	7.0	4.0	15
sauce, ranch	1 serving	170	17.0	0.0	2.0	1.0	0
sauce, tartar	1 serving	180	19.0	0.0	0.0	0.0	15
shake, chocolate	1 medium	320	7.0	9.0	54.0	48.0	20
shake, strawberry	1 medium	420	6.0	9.0	83.0	78.0	20
shake, vanilla	1 medium	300	6.0	9.0	53.0	47.0	20
Whopper sandwich	1 sandwich	640	39.0	27.0	45.0	8.0	90
Whopper, double	1 sandwich	870	56.0	46.0	45.0	8.0	170
Whopper, double with cheese	1 sandwich	960	63.0	52.0	46.0	8.0	195
Whopper, Jr.	1 sandwich	420	24.0	21.0	29.0	5.0	60
Whopper, Jr., with cheese	1 sandwich	460	28.0	23.0	29.0	5.0	75
Whopper, with cheese	1 sandwich	730	46.0	33.0	46.0	8.0	115
DAIRY QUEEN							
banana split	regular	510	12	8	96	82	30
buster bar	1 bar	450	28	10	41	33	15
Butterfinger blizzard	regular	750	26	16	115	92	50
chocolate cone	regular	360	11	9	56	37	30

Food	Portion	Calories	Fat	Protein	Carb	Sugar	Chol
chocolate dilly bar	1 bar	450	28	3	21	17	15
chocolate malt	regular	880	22	19	153	131	70
chocolate mint dilly bar	1 bar	190	12	3	20	20	15
chocolate rock treat	regular	730	38				30
chocolate shake	regular	770	20	17	130	113	70
chocolate sundae	regular	410	10	8	73	63	30
cone, dipped	regular	510	25	9	63	46	30
cookie dough blizzard	regular	950	36	17	142	106	75
DQ caramel nut bar	1 bar	260	13	5	32	32	15
DQ fudge bar	1 bar	50	0	4	13	3	0
DQ orange bar	1 bar	60	0				0
DQ sandwich	regular	150	5	3	24	13	5
DQ chocolate soft serve	½ cup	150	5	4	22	17	15
DQ frozen heart cake	1 slice	270	9	5	41	30	20
DQ frozen log cake	1 slice	280	9	5	43	31	15
DQ frozen round cake	1 slice	340	12	7	53	39	25
DQ frozen sheet cake	1 slice	350	12	7	54	39	20
DQ lemon Freez'r	½ cup	80	0	0	20	20	0
DQ nonfat frozen yogurt	½ cup	100	0	3	21	16	0
DQ vanilla orange bar	1 bar	60	0	2	17	2	0
DQ vanilla soft serve	½ cup	140	5	3	22	19	15
fudge cake supreme	regular	890	38				65
fudge nut bar	1 bar	410	25	8	40	33	15
Heath blizzard	regular	820	33	14	119	106	60
Heath breeze	regular	710	18	15	123	103	20

Food	Portion	Calories	Fat	Protein	Carb	Sugar	Chol
Heath DQ Treatzza Pizza	1 slice	180	7	3	28	18	5
misty slush	regular	290	0	0	74	74	0
M&M DQ Treatzza Pizza	1 slice	190	7	3	29	20	5
Oreo blizzard	regular	640	23	10	79	61	45
peanut buster parfait	regular	730	31	16	99	85	35
peanut butter fudge DQ Treatzza Pizza	1 slice	220	10	4	28	18	5
Queen's Choice chocolate big scoop	regular	250	14	4	28	24	55
Queen's Choice vanilla big scoop	regular	250	14	4	27	22	55
Reese's Peanut Butter Cup blizzard	regular	790	33	19	105	88	55
starkiss	regular	80	0	0	21	21	0
strawberry-banana DQ Treatzza Pizza	1 slice	180	6	3	29	19	5
strawberry blizzard	regular	570	16	12	95	82	50
strawberry breeze	regular	460	1	13	99	79	10
strawberry misty cooler	regular	190	0	0	49	49	0
strawberry shortcake	regular	430	14	7	24	13	60
toffee dilly bar	1 bar	210	12	3	24	17	15
vanilla cone	regular	350	10	8	57	41	30
yogurt cup	regular	230	1	8	49	38	5
yogurt cone	regular	280	1	9	59	39	5
yogurt strawberry sundae	regular	300	1	10	66	53	5
DENNY'S							
apple pie	7 oz	470	24	3	64	36	0
banana split	19 oz	894	43	15	121	29	78

Food	Portion	Calories	Fat	Protein	Carb	Sugar	Chol
biscuit, sausage gravy	7 oz	398	21	8	45	0	12
buffalo wings	12 pieces	856	54	92	1	0	500
carrots, honey glaze	4 oz	80	3	1	12	7	0
Charleston chicken dinner	6 oz	327	18	25	16	0	65
cheesecake pie	4 oz	470	27	6	48	31	90
cheese fries, chili	12 oz	816	44	29	77	4	74
cheese fries, smothered	9 oz	767	48	27	69	1	78
cherry pie	7 oz	630	25	3	101	64	0
chicken burger	1 sandwich	632	32	35	53	6	81
chicken burger, buffalo	1 sandwich	803	45	37	67	8	77
chicken-fried steak	4 oz	265	17	15	14	0	27
chicken strips	5 pieces	720	33	47	56	14	95
chicken strips, buffalo	5 pieces	734	42	48	43	0	96
chili, cheese topping	11 oz	401	19	26	21	9	57
chocolate layer cake	3 oz	275	12	4	42	24	26
chocolate peanut butter pie	6 oz	653	39	15	64	45	27
club sandwich	1 sandwich	718	38	32	62	6	75
corn, butter sauce	4 oz	120	4	3	19	4	5
country-fried potatoes	6 oz	515	35	3	23	0	8
double-scoop sundae	6 oz	375	27	6	29	8	74
french fries	4 oz	323	14	5	44	0	0
french fries, seasoned	4 oz	261	12	5	35	0	0
fried shrimp dinner	8 oz	219	10	17	18	5	133
garden salad deluxe with chicken	14 oz	264	11	32	10	5	89

Food	Portion	Calories	Fat	Protein	Carb	Sugar	Chol
grasshopper blender blaster	15 oz	735	37	13	92	86	140
grasshopper sundae	14 oz	734	34	13	97	84	97
green beans, bacon	4 oz	60	4	1	6	2	5
green peas, butter sauce	4 oz	100	2	5	14	6	5
grilled chicken dinner	4 oz	130	4	24	0	0	67
grilled chicken sandwich	1 sandwich	434	9	35	56	11	82
grilled chicken stir-fry	19 oz	864	10	43	149	15	67
grilled salmon dinner	6 oz	210	4	43	1	0	101
ham, Swiss sandwich	1 sandwich	533	31	23	40	9	36
hamburger, bacon cheddar	1 sandwich	875	52	53	58	9	163
hamburger, Big Texas BBQ	1 sandwich	929	58	53	53	8	163
hamburger, boca	1 sandwich	616	28	29	66	10	14
hamburger, classic	1 sandwich	673	40	37	42	7	106
hamburger, classic doubledecker	1 sandwich	1377	92	62	81	10	210
hamburger, classic with cheese	1 sandwich	836	53	47	43	7	137
hamburger, mushroom Swiss	1 sandwich	872	51	48	58	9	116
Hershey's chocolate chip pie	5.5 oz	600	36	6	58	42	10
hot fudge cake sundae	7 oz	620	35	7	73	43	60
malted milk shake, chocolate	12 oz	583	26	12	82	71	100
malted milk shake, vanilla	12 oz	583	26	12	82	71	100
mashed potatoes	6 oz	105	1	3	21	1	0

Food	Portion	Calories	Fat	Protein	Carb	Sugar	Chol
mashed potatoes, cheddar	6 oz	117	2	3	22	1	2
mozzarella sticks	8 pieces	710	41	36	49	0	48
onion rings	4 oz	381	23	5	38	2	6
Oreo cookies and creme pie	6 oz	651	40	6	67	47	20
peaches and cream sundae	10 oz	568	22	5	91	78	81
pot roast dinner	7 oz	292	11	42	5	0	87
roast turkey dinner	14 oz	388	3	46	38	17	116
Rueben sandwich	1 sandwich	580	35	27	37	10	69
shake, chocolate	12 oz	560	26	11	76	71	100
shake, vanilla	12 oz	560	26	11	76	71	100
shrimp scampi skillet dinner	5 oz	289	19	25	3	0	192
sirloin steak dinner	8 oz	337	28	18	1	0	687
Slim Slam	12 oz	495	12	34	98	7	34
steak and shrimp dinner	9 oz	645	42	36	31	4	150
Super Bird sandwich	1 sandwich	620	32	35	48	4	60
T-bone steak dinner	14 oz	860	65	65	0	0	196
two-egg breakfast	11 oz	825	67	6	1	0	538
turkey breast sandwich	1 sandwich	476	26	23	39	5	57
vegetable rice pilaf	3 oz	85	1	2	16	0	0
Western wing roundup	20 oz	1517	88	89	89	9	465
DOMINO'S PIZZA							
cheese pizza	2 slices	344	10	14.8	50.0	1.0	19
cheese deep-dish pizza	2 slices	560	24	11.5	63.2	4.3	32

Food	Portion	Calories	Fat	Protein	Carb	Sugar	Chol
cheese, pepperoni pizza	2 slices	455	19	20.9	50.5	1.0	42
cheese, pepperoni deep-dish pizza	2 slices	622	33	29.6	63.7	4.4	54
ham pizza	2 slices	362	10	17.2	50.3	1.2	26
ham deep-dish pizza	2 slices	577	25	25.9	63.5	4.5	38
Italian sausage pizza	2 slices	402	14	17.5	52.2	1.3	31
Italian sausage deep-dish pizza	2 slices	678	28	26.9	65.5	4.6	43
pepperoni pizza	2 slices	406	15	17.5	50.2	1.0	32
pepperoni deep-dish pizza	2 slices	622	29	26.2	63.4	4.4	45
DUNKIN' DONUTS							
apple crumb	1 donut	230	10	3	34	12	0
apple fritter	1 donut	300	14	4	41	12	0
banana nut	1 muffin	530	23	10	72	37	70
Bavarian kreme	1 donut	210	9	3	30	9	0
biscuit, bacon, cheddar	1 sandwich	500	290	21	33	4	300
biscuit, egg, cheese	1 sandwich	380	22	17	30	3	180
biscuit, sausage, egg, cheese	1 sandwich	590	42	25	31	4	220
blueberry	1 muffin	490	17	8	76	41	75
blueberry cake donut	1 donut	290	16	3	35	16	10
Boston kreme	1 donut	240	9	3	36	14	0
bow tie	1 donut	300	17	4	34	10	0
butternut cake ring	1 donut	300	16	3	36	16	0
cake Munchkin, cinnamon	4 Munchkins	250	14	3	30	13	0
cake Munchkin, plain	4 Munchkins	220	14	2	22	6	0

Food	Portion	Calories	Fat	Protein	Carb	Sugar	Chol
cake Munchkin, powdered	4 Munchkins	250	14	2	29	12	0
chocolate coconut cake	1 donut	300	19	4	31	12	0
chocolate frosted coffee roll	1 donut	290	15	4	36	12	0
chocolate glazed cake	1 donut	290	16	3	33	14	0
cinnamon bun	1 bun	510	15	8	85	42	10
cinnamon cake	1 donut	270	15	3	31	12	0
coconut cake	1 donut	290	17	3	33	13	0
corn	1 muffin	500	16	10	78	34	80
cruller, glazed	1 donut	290	15	3	37	18	0
cruller, plain	1 donut	240	15	3	25	6	0
Dunkin' Donut	1 donut	240	15	3	25	17	0
eclair	1 donut	270	11	3	39	17	0
fritter, glazed	1 donut	260	14	4	31	7	0
glazed	1 donut	180	8	3	25	6	0
glazed cake	1 donut	270	15	3	33	14	0
jelly-filled	1 donut	210	8	3	32	14	0
lemon poppyseed	1 muffin	580	19	10	94	53	85
old-fashioned cake	1 donut	250	15	3	26	7	0
Omwich, bagel, bacon, cheddar	1 sandwich	600	21	26	79	5	295
Omwich, bagel pizza	1 sandwich	560	19	25	74	5	255
Omwich, bagel, Spanish	1 sandwich	570	18	24	79	5	280
Omwich, croissant, bacon, cheddar	1 sandwich	560	38	21	33	5	295
Omwich, croissant pizza	1 sandwich	510	34	18	33	6	260
yeast Munchkin, glazed	5 Munchkins	200	9	3	27	12	0
yeast Munchkin, sugar	7 Munchkins	220	12	4	26	5	0

Food	Portion	Calories	Fat	Protein	Carb	Sugar	Chol
HARDEE'S							
baked beans	5 oz	170	1.0	8.0	32.0		0
cookie	2 oz	280	12.0	4.0	41.0		15
Big Country Breakfast, bacon	1 serving	820	49.0	33.0	62.0		535
Big Country Breakfast, sausage	1 serving	1000	66.0	41.0	62.0		570
biscuit, apple	1 biscuit	200	8.0	2.0	30.0		0
biscuit, bacon, egg	1 biscuit	570	33.0	22.0	45.0		275
biscuit, bacon, egg, cheese	1 biscuit	610	37.0	24.0	45.0		260
biscuit, country ham	1 biscuit	430	22.0	15.0	45.0		25
biscuit, gravy	1 biscuit	510	28.0	10.0	55.0		15
biscuit, sausage	1 biscuit	510	31.0	14.0	44.0		25
cheeseburger	1 sandwich	310	14.0	6.0			40
cheeseburger, mesquite bacon	1 sandwich	370	18.0	19.0	32.0		45
cheeseburger, Quarter-Pound Double	1 sandwich	470	27.0	27.0	31.0		80
chicken fillet sandwich	1 sandwich	480	18.0	26.0	54.0		55
chicken, fried, breast	1 piece	370	15.0	29.0	29.0		75
chicken, fried, leg	1 piece	170	7.0	13.0	15.0		45
chicken, grilled sandwich	1 sandwich	350	11.0	25.0	38.0		65
Fisherman's Fillet sandwich	1 sandwich	560	27.0	26.0	54.0		65
french fries	large	430	18.0	6.0	58.0		0
french fries	medium	350	15.0	5.0	48.0		0
french fries	small	240	10.0	4.0	33.0		0
Frisco breakfast sandwich, ham	1 sandwich	500	25.0	24.0	46.0		290
hamburger	1 sandwich	270	11.0	14.0	29.0		35
hamburger, Frisco	1 sandwich	720	46.0	33.0	43.0		95
hamburger, The Boss	1 sandwich	570	33.0	27.0	42.0		85

Food	Portion	Calories	Fat	Protein	Carb	Sugar	Chol
hamburger, The Works	1 sandwich	530	30.0	25.0	41.0		80
hash rounds	1 serving	230	14.0	3.0	24.0		0
ham and cheese sandwich, hot	1 sandwich	310	12.0	18.0	34.0		50
pancakes	3 pancakes	280	2.0	8.0	56.0		15
peach cobbler	1 cobbler	310	7.0	2.0	60.0		0
roast beef sandwich	1 sandwich	320	18.0	17.0	26.0		48
roast beef sandwich, big	1 sandwich	460	24.0	26.0	35.0		70
salad, grilled chicken	1 salad	150	3.0	20.0	11.0		60
shake, chocolate	1 shake	370	5.0	13.0	67.0		30
shake, peach	1 shake	390	4.0	10.0	77.0		25
shake, strawberry	1 shake	420	4.0	11.0	83.0		20
shake, vanilla	1 shake	350	5.0	12.0	65.0		20
sundae, hot fudge	1 sundae	290	6.0	7.0	51.0		20
sundae, strawberry	1 sundae	210	2.0	5.0	43.0		10
JACK-IN-THE-BOX							
Breakfast Jack	1 sandwich	300	12	18.0	30.0	5.0	185
cake, carrot	1 slice	370	15	3.0	58.0	39.0	80
cheeseburger	1 sandwich	320	15	16.0	32.0	5.0	35
cheeseburger, double	1 sandwich	450	24	24.0	35.0	6.0	75
cheeseburger, ultimate	1 sandwich	1,030	79	50.0	30.0	6.0	205
cheesecake	1 slice	310	18	8.0	29.0	22.0	65
chicken fajita pita	1 sandwich	290	8.0	24.0	29.0	3.0	35
chicken strips	6 pieces	450	20.0	39.0	28.0	0.0	80
chicken teriyaki bowl	1 bowl	580	1.5	28.0	115.0	20.0	55
egg rolls	5 pieces	750	41	5.0	92.0	10.0	50
french fries	jumbo	400	19	5.0	51.0	0.0	0
french fries	regular	350	17	4.0	45.0	0.0	0
french fries	small	220	11	3.0	28.0	0.0	0

Food	Portion	Calories	Fat	Protein	Carb	Sugar	Chol
french fries	super	590	29	8.0	76.0	0.0	0
french fries, curly	regular	360	20	5.0	39.0	0.0	0
hamburger	1 sandwich	280	11	13.0	31.0	5.0	25
hash browns	2 oz	160	11	1.0	14.0	0.0	0
jalapenos, stuffed	10 pieces	600	39	22.0	41.0	4.0	75
Jumbo Jack	1 sandwich	560	32	26.0	41.0	6.0	65
Jumbo Jack, cheese	1 sandwich	650	40	31.0	42.0	6.0	90
onion rings	medium	380	23	5.0	38.0	4.0	0
pancake platter	1 platter	400	12.0	13.0	59.0	12.0	30
potato wedges, bacon, cheddar	1 serving	800	58.0	20.0	49.0	2.0	55
sandwich, chicken	1 sandwich	400	18	20.0	38.0	0.0	45
sandwich, chicken caesar	1 sandwich	520	26	27.0	44.0	5.0	55
sandwich, chicken supreme	1 sandwich	620	36	25.0	48.0	5.0	75
sandwich, grilled chicken	1 sandwich	430	19	29.0	36.0	7.0	65
sandwich, spicy chicken	1 sandwich	560	27	24.0	55.0	5.0	50
sausage croissant	1 sandwich	670	48.0	21.0	39.0	4.0	250
scrambled egg pocket	1 sandwich	430	21.0	29.0	31.0	0.0	355
shake, cappuccino	1 shake	630	29	11.0	80.0	58.0	90
shake, chocolate	1 shake	630	27	11.0	85.0	67.0	85
shake, strawberry	1 shake	640	28	10.0	85.0	67.0	85
shake, vanilla	1 shake	610	31	12.0	73.0	12.0	95
sourdough breakfast sandwich	1 sandwich	380	20.0	21.0	31.0	2.0	235
supreme croissant	1 sandwich	570	36.0	21.0	39.0	4.0	245
taco	1 taco	190	11	7.0	15.0	0.0	20
taco, monster	1 taco	283	17	12.0	22.0	1.0	30

KENTUCKY FRIED CHICKEN (KFC)

Food	Portion	Calories	Fat	Protein	Carb	Sugar	Chol
baked beans, BBQ	5 oz	190	3	6.0	33.0	13.0	5
biscuit	1 biscuit	180	10	4.0	20.0	2.0	0

Food	Portion	Calories	Fat	Protein	Carb	Sugar	Chol
chicken, extra tasty crispy	breast	470	28	31.0	25.0	0.0	80
chicken, extra tasty crispy	leg	190	11	13.0	8.0	0.0	60
chicken, extra tasty crispy	thigh	370	25	19.0	18.0	0.0	70
chicken, extra tasty crispy	wing	200	13	10.0	10.0	0.0	45
chicken, hot and spicy	breast	530	35	32.0	23.0	0.0	110
chicken, hot and spicy	leg	190	11	13.0	10.0	0.0	50
chicken, hot and spicy	thigh	370	27	18.0	13.0	0.0	90
chicken, hot and spicy	wing	210	15	10.0	9.0	0.0	50
chicken, original recipe	breast	400	24	29.0	16.0	0.0	135
chicken, original recipe	leg	140	9	13.0	4.0	0.0	75
chicken, original recipe	thigh	250	18	16.0	6.0	0.0	95
chicken, original recipe	wing	140	10	9.0	5.0	0.0	55
chicken sandwich, BBQ	1 sandwich	256	8	17.0	28.0	18.0	57
chicken sandwich, original recipe	1 sandwich	497	22.3	28.6	45.5	2.0	52
chicken, tender roast	breast	251	10.8	37.0	1.0	0.0	151
chicken, tender roast	leg	97	4.3	14.5	0.0	0.0	85
chicken, tender roast	thigh	207	12	18.4	0.0	0.0	120
chicken, tender roast	wing	121	7.7	12.2	1.0	0.0	74
chunky chicken pot pie	1 pie	770	42.0	29.0	69.0	8.0	70
coleslaw	5 oz	180	9.0	2.0	21.0	20.0	5

Food	Portion	Calories	Fat	Protein	Carb	Sugar	Chol
Colonel's Crispy Strips	3 strips	261	15.8	19.8	10.0	0.0	40
cornbread	1 piece	228	13	3.0	25.0	10.0	42
Hot Wings	6 pieces	471	33	27.0	18.0	0.0	150
Kentucky Nuggets	medium	284	18	16.0	15.0	0.0	66
macaroni and cheese	medium	180	8	7.0	21.0	2.0	10
Mean Greens	medium	70	3	4.0	11.0	1.0	10
potato salad	6 oz	230	14.0	4.0	23.0	9.0	15
potato wedges	5 oz	280	13.0	5.0	28.0	1.0	5
potatoes, mashed	medium	120	6	1.0	17.0	0.0	0
red beans and rice	medium	130	3	5.0	21.0	2.0	5

LONG JOHN SILVER'S

Food	Portion	Calories	Fat	Protein	Carb	Sugar	Chol
cheesesticks	3 pieces	160	9	6	12		10
chicken, battered plank	1 piece	140	8	8	9		20
chicken sandwich	1 sandwich	340	14	13	40		25
chicken sandwich, cheese	1 sandwich	390	19	16	40		40
clam chowder	bowl	520	24	24	52		70
clams, breaded	1 order	250	14	9	26		35
cole slaw	4 oz	170	7	2	23		0
crabcake	1 cake	150	9	4	12		15
fish, battered	1 piece	230	13	12	16		30
fish, battered, junior	1 piece	120	8	5	8		15
fish, country breaded	1 piece	200	10	10	17		10
fish, lemon crumb	2 pieces	240	12	23	10		4
fish sandwich	1 sandwich	430	20	16	46		35
fish sandwich, cheese	1 sandwich	480	25	19	46		50
fish sandwich, ultimate	1 sandwich	480	25	19	46		50
french fries	regular	250	15	3	28		0
french fries	large	420	24	5	46		0

Food	Portion	Calories	Fat	Protein	Carb	Sugar	Chol
hushpuppy	1 piece	60	3	9	25		0
pie, banana split sundae	1 piece	300	17	4	34		15
pie, chocolate creme	1 piece	280	17	4	29		15
pie, Dutch apple	1 piece	290	13	2	44		0
pie, pecan	1 piece	390	19	3	53		40
pie, pineapple creme cheesecake	1 piece	310	17	4	36		5
pie, strawberries, cream	1 piece	280	15	4	32		15
salad, grilled chicken	1 salad	140	3	10	20		45
salad, ocean chef	1 salad	130	2	14	15		60
shrimp, battered	1 piece	45	3	2	3		15
shrimp, popcorn	1 serving	320	15	15	33		85

MCDONALD'S

Food	Portion	Calories	Fat	Protein	Carb	Sugar	Chol
Big Mac	1 sandwich	560	32.4	25.2	42.5		103
biscuit	1 biscuit	260	12.7	3.4	8.6	0.6	1
biscuit, bacon, egg, cheese	1 biscuit	440	26.4	17.5	33.3		253
biscuit, sausage	1 biscuit	440	29	13.0	31.9		49
biscuit, sausage, egg	1 biscuit	520	34.5	19.9	32.6		275
cheeseburger	1 sandwich	310	13.8	15.0	31.2		53
chicken McNuggets	1 serving	290	16.3	19.0	16.5		65
cookies, Chocolaty Chip	1 box	330	15.6	4.2	41.9		4
cookies, McDonaldland	1 box	290	9.2	4.2	47.1		10
Danish, apple	1 Danish	390	17.9	5.8	51.2		25
Danish, cheese	1 Danish	390	21.8	7.4	42.3		47
Danish, cinnamon	1 Danish	440	21	6.4	57.5		34
Danish, raspberry	1 Danish	410	15.9	6.1	61.5		26
Egg McMuffin	1 sandwich	290	11.2	18.2	28.1		226
Fillet-o-Fish sandwich	1 sandwich	440	26.1	13.8	37.9		50

Food	Portion	Calories	Fat	Protein	Carb	Sugar	Chol
french fries	large	400	21.6	5.6	45.9		16
french fries	medium	320	17.1	4.4	36.3		12
french fries	small	220	12	3.1	25.6		9
frozen yogurt hot caramel sundae	1 sundae	270	2.8	6.6	59.3		13
frozen yogurt hot fudge sundae	1 sundae	240	3.2	7.3	50.5		6
frozen yogurt strawberry sundae	1 sundae	210	1.1	5.7	49.2		5
frozen yogurt vanilla cone	1 cone	100	0.8	4.0	22.0		3
hamburger	1 sandwich	260	9.5	12.2	30.6		37
hash brown potatoes	1 serving	130	7.3	1.4	14.9		9
hotcakes, butter, syrup	1 serving	410	9.2	8.2	74.4		21
McChicken	1 sandwich	490	28.6	19.2	39.8		43
pie, apple	1 pie	260	14.8	2.2	30.0		6
Quarter Pounder	1 sandwich	410	20.7	23.1	34.0		86
Quarter Pounder, cheese	1 sandwich	520	29.2	28.5	35.1		118
salad, chef	1 salad	230	13.3	20.5	7.5		128
salad, chunky chicken	1 salad	140	3.4	23.1	5.3		78
salad, garden	1 salad	110	6.6	7.1	6.2		83
sausage McMuffin	1 sandwich	370	21.9	16.5	27.3		64
sausage McMuffin, egg	1 sandwich	440	26.8	22.6	27.9		263
shake, chocolate	1 shake	320	1.7	11.6	66.0		10
shake, strawberry	1 shake	320	1.3	10.7	67.0		10
shake, vanilla	1 shake	290	1.3	10.8	60.0		10
PIZZA HUT							
apple dessert pizza	1 slice	250	4.5	3	48	25	0
bread stick	1 serving	130	4	3	20	1	0
cavatini pasta	1 serving	480	14	21	66	12	8

Food	Portion	Calories	Fat	Protein	Carb	Sugar	Chol
cavatini supreme pasta	1 serving	560	19	24	73	11	10
cherry dessert pizza	1 slice	250	4.5	3	47	24	0
Bigfoot pizza, cheese	1 slice	186	6	10	25	1	16
Bigfoot pizza, pepperoni	1 slice	205	7	10	25	2	20
buffalo wings, hot	4 pieces	210	12	22	4	0	130
buffalo wings, mild	5 pieces	200	12	23	0	0	150
garlic bread	1 slice	150	8	3	16	0	0
Hand Tossed pizza, beef	1 slice	260	9	16	29	1	26
Hand Tossed pizza, cheese	1 slice	235	7	12	28	1	25
Hand Tossed pizza, ham	1 slice	213	5	14	28	1	21
Hand Tossed pizza, pepperoni	1 slice	238	8	13	28	2	24
Hand Tossed pizza, sausage	1 slice	267	11	16	28	2	31
Hand Tossed pizza, supreme	1 slice	284	12	13	29	2	30
Pan Pizza, beef	1 slice	286	13	14	28	1	26
Pan Pizza, cheese	1 slice	261	11	12	28	1	25
Pan Pizza, ham	1 slice	239	9	11	28	2	21
Pan Pizza, pepperoni	1 slice	265	12	11	28	2	24
Pan Pizza, supreme	1 slice	311	15	15	28	2	30
Pan Pizza, veggie	1 slice	243	10	10	29	2	17
spaghetti, marinara sauce	1 serving	490	6	18	91	10	0
spaghetti, meat sauce	1 serving	600	13	23	98	10	8
spaghetti, meatballs	1 serving	850	24	37	120	12	17

Food	Portion	Calories	Fat	Protein	Carb	Sugar	Chol
Stuffed Crust pizza, beef	1 slice	466	22	23	46	1	30
Stuffed Crust pizza, cheese	1 slice	445	19	22	46	1	24
Stuffed Crust pizza, ham	1 slice	404	22	24	45	3	39
Stuffed Crust pizza, pepperoni	1 slice	438	19	21	45	1	27
Stuffed Crust pizza, sausage	1 slice	478	23	22	46	1	35
Thin 'n Crispy Pizza, beef	1 slice	229	11	13	22	1	26
Thin 'n Crispy Pizza, cheese	1 slice	205	8	10	22	1	25
Thin 'n Crispy Pizza, ham	1 slice	184	7	9	21	1	22
Thin 'n Crispy Pizza, pepperoni	1 slice	215	10	9	21	1	25
Thin 'n Crispy Pizza, sausage	1 slice	236	12	12	22	1	31
Thin 'n Crispy Pizza, supreme	1 slice	257	13	12	23	2	31
Thin 'n Crispy Pizza, veggie	1 slice	186	7	8	24	3	17
SUBWAY							
Berry Lishus drink	small	113	0	0	28	27	0
breakfast sandwich, bacon, egg	6" sandwich	305	15	13	29	3	184
breakfast sandwich, cheese, egg	6" sandwich	302	15	13	29	3	187
breakfast sandwich, ham, egg	6" sandwich	291	12	15	30	4	189
breakfast sandwich, western	6" sandwich	285	12	13	31	3	182
classic salad, BMT	1 salad	272	19	16	11	1	56

Food	Portion	Calories	Fat	Protein	Carb	Sugar	Chol
classic salad, cold cut trio	1 salad	234	15	14	11	1	57
classic salad, meatball	1 salad	320	20	17	17	2	56
classic salad, seafood and crab	1 salad	197	11	9	17	1	24
classic salad, steak and cheese	1 salad	181	8	17	12	2	37
classic salad, Subway melt	1 salad	203	10	17	11	1	44
classic salad, tuna	1 salad	238	16	13	10	0	42
classic sandwich, BMT	6" sandwich	453	24	21	40	5	56
classic sandwich, cold cut trio	6" sandwich	415	20	19	40	5	57
classic sandwich, meatball	6" sandwich	501	25	23	46	7	56
classic sandwich, seafood and crab	6" sandwich	378	16	14	46	6	24
classic sandwich, steak and cheese	6" sandwich	362	13	23	41	7	37
classic sandwich, Subway melt	6" sandwich	384	15	22	40	6	44
classic sandwich, tuna	6" sandwich	419	21	18	39	5	42
cookie, chocolate chip	1 cookie	209	10	3	29	17	12
cookie, chocolate chunk	1 cookie	210	10	2	30	17	12
cookie, M&M	1 cookie	210	10	2	29	17	13
cookie, oatmeal raisin	1 cookie	197	8	3	29	17	14
cookie, peanut butter	1 cookie	220	12	3	26	14	0
cookie, sugar	1 cookie	222	12	2	28	14	18
cookie, white macadamia nut	1 cookie	221	12	2	27	15	13
deli sandwich, ham	6" sandwich	194	4	10	30	3	12

Food	Portion	Calories	Fat	Protein	Carb	Sugar	Chol
deli sandwich, roast beef	6" sandwich	206	4	12	31	3	13
deli sandwich, tuna	6" sandwich	309	15	12	31	2	26
deli sandwich, turkey breast	6" sandwich	200	4	12	31	2	13
Peach Pizazz drink	small	103	0	0	26	26	0
Pineapple Delight drink	small	133	0	1	33	33	0
select sandwich, caesar chicken	6" sandwich	391	15	22	41	6	47
select sandwich, Italian BMT	6" sandwich	530	31	22	41	6	66
select sandwich, honey mustard melt	6" sandwich	376	11	22	47	11	44
select sandwich, honey mustard turkey	6" sandwich	275	4	16	46	11	20
select sandwich, roast beef	6" sandwich	401	17	18	42	8	27
select sandwich, steak and cheese	6" sandwich	468	22	22	43	9	44
select sandwich, southwest chicken	6" sandwich	362	13	21	40	7	43
select sandwich, southwest steak	6" sandwich	412	18	22	42	8	44
7 under 6 sandwich, ham	6" sandwich	261	5	17	39	6	25
7 under 6 sandwich, roast beef	6" sandwich	264	5	18	39	6	20
7 under 6 sandwich, chicken breast	6" sandwich	311	6	25	40	5	48
7 under 6 sandwich, Subway club	6" sandwich	294	5	22	40	6	33

Food	Portion	Calories	Fat	Protein	Carb	Sugar	Chol
7 under 6 sandwich, turkey breast	6" sandwich	254	4	16	39	5	20
7 under 6 sandwich, turkey and ham	6" sandwich	267	5	18	40	5	26
7 under 6 sandwich, veggie delite	6" sandwich	200	3	7	37	4	0
Sunrise Refresher drink	small	119	0	1	29	28	0
wrap, caesar chicken	6" sandwich	413	15	22	47	3	47
wrap, steak and cheese	6" sandwich	353	9	22	46	3	37
wrap, turkey breast and bacon	6" sandwich	321	7	18	45	2	28
TACO BELL							
burrito, bean	1 burrito	370	12	13	54	3	10
burrito, beef fiesta	1 burrito	380	15	14	49	3	30
burrito, beef supreme	1 burrito	420	18	17	50	4	40
burrito, chicken fiesta	1 burrito	370	12	17	48	2	35
burrito, chicken supreme	1 burrito	410	16	20	49	4	30
burrito, chili cheese	1 burrito	330	13	13	40	2	25
burrito, double beef supreme	1 burrito	510	23	23	52	4	60
burrito, double chicken supreme	1 burrito	460	17	27	50	4	70
burrito, double steak supreme	1 burrito	470	18	28	48	3	55
burrito, grilled beef	1 burrito	730	35	27	75	4	65

Food	Portion	Calories	Fat	Protein	Carb	Sugar	Chol
burrito, grilled chicken	1 burrito	690	29	33	73	4	70
burrito, grilled steak	1 burrito	690	30	30	72	4	60
burrito, seven-layer	1 burrito	520	22	16	65	4	25
burrito, steak fiesta	1 burrito	370	12	18	47	2	25
burrito, steak supreme	1 burrito	420	16	21	48	4	35
chalupa baja, beef	1 chalupa	420	27	14	30	3	35
chalupa baja, chicken	1 chalupa	400	24	17	28	3	40
chalupa baja, steak	1 chalupa	400	24	17	27	3	30
chalupa, beef supreme	1 chalupa	380	23	14	29	3	40
chalupa, chicken supreme	1 chalupa	360	20	17	28	3	45
chalupa nacho cheese, beef	1 chalupa	370	22	13	30	3	25
chalupa nacho cheese, chicken	1 chalupa	350	19	16	29	3	25
chalupa nacho cheese, steak	1 chalupa	350	19	16	28	2	20
chalupa Santa Fe, beef	1 chalupa	440	29	14	31	2	35
chalupa Santa Fe, chicken	1 chalupa	420	26	17	30	2	40
chalupa Santa Fe, steak	1 chalupa	430	27	18	29	2	35
chalupa, steak supreme	1 chalupa	360	20	17	27	3	35
cinnamon twists	1 serving	150	7	1	27	13	0
enchirito, beef	1 enchirito	370	19	18	33	2	50
enchirito, chicken	1 enchirito	350	16	21	32	2	55
enchirito, steak	1 enchirito	350	16	22	31	2	45
gordita baja, beef	1 gordita	360	21	13	29	4	35

Food	Portion	Calories	Fat	Protein	Carb	Sugar	Chol
gordita baja, chicken	1 gordita	340	18	16	28	4	40
gordita baja, steak	1 gordita	340	18	15	28	3	35
gordita, beef supreme	1 gordita	300	14	17	27	4	35
gordita, cheesy crunch	1 gordita	560	33	21	44	4	60
gordita, cheesy crunch supreme	1 gordita	610	37	22	47	5	70
gordita, chicken supreme	1 gordita	300	13	16	28	3	45
gordita, nacho cheese, beef	1 gordita	310	15	13	30	4	25
gordita, nacho cheese, chicken	1 gordita	290	13	15	29	4	25
gordita, nacho cheese, steak	1 gordita	290	13	16	28	3	20
gordita Santa Fe, beef	1 gordita	380	23	14	31	3	35
gordita Santa Fe, chicken	1 gordita	370	20	17	30	3	40
gordita Santa Fe, steak	1 gordita	370	20	17	29	3	35
gordita, steak supreme	1 gordita	300	14	17	27	3	35
Mexican pizza	1 pizza	390	25	18	28	2	45
Mexican rice	1 serving	190	13	5	23	0	15
MexiMelt	1 serving	290	15	15	22	2	45
nachos	1 serving	320	18	5	34	2	5
nachos BellGrande	1 serving	760	39	20	83	4	35
nachos supreme	1 serving	440	24	14	44	3	35
pintos, cheese	1 serving	180	8	9	18	1	15
quesadilla, cheese	1 quesadilla	350	18	16	31	2	50
quesadilla, chicken	1 quesadilla	400	19	25	33	2	75
taco	1 taco	210	12	9	18	0	30
taco, double decker	1 taco	380	17	15	43	2	15

Food	Portion	Calories	Fat	Protein	Carb	Sugar	Chol
taco, double decker supreme	1 taco	420	21	15	45	3	40
taco, soft, beef	1 taco	210	10	11	20	1	30
taco, soft, chicken	1 taco	190	7	13	19	1	35
taco, soft, steak	1 taco	280	17	12	20	2	35
taco, Supreme	1 taco	260	16	10	20	2	40
taco salad	1 salad	850	52	30	69	12	70
tostada	1 tostada	250	12	10	27	2	15
WENDY'S							
baked potato, bacon, cheese	1	530	18	17	78	5	25
baked potato, broccoli, cheese	1	470	14	9	80	6	5
baked potato, cheese	1	570	23	14	78	5	30
baked potato, chili, cheese	1	620	24	20	83	7	40
baked potato, sour cream, chive	1	370	5	7	73	6	20
cheeseburger, bacon, junior	1 sandwich	390	20	20	34	7	55
cheeseburger, deluxe junior	1 sandwich	360	17	18	36	8	50
cheeseburger, junior	1 sandwich	320	13	17	34	7	45
cheeseburger, kids' meal	1 meal	320	13	17	34	7	45
chicken nuggets	5 pieces	190	13	9	9	0	25
chicken sandwich, breaded	1 sandwich	440	18	28	44	6	60
chicken sandwich, club	1 sandwich	480	21	30	44	6	65
chicken sandwich, grilled	1 sandwich	300	8	24	36	8	55
chicken sandwich, spicy	1 sandwich	410	15	28	43	6	65
chili	large	310	10	23	32	8	45
chili	small	310	7	15	21	5	45

Food	Portion	Calories	Fat	Protein	Carb	Sugar	Chol
cookies, chocolate chip	1 cookie	270	13	3	36	16	30
dairy dessert, Frosty	large	540	14	14	91	70	60
dairy dessert, Frosty	medium	440	11	11	73	56	50
dairy dessert, Frosty	small	330	8	8	56	43	35
french fries	biggie	470	23	7	61	0	0
french fries	super	570	27	8	73	0	0
french fries	small	270	13	4	35	0	0
hamburger, big bacon classic	1 sandwich	580	31	33	45	11	95
hamburger, classic single	1 sandwich	360	16	24	31	5	65
hamburger, classic single, everything	1 sandwich	420	20	25	37	8	70
hamburger, junior	1 sandwich	280	10	15	34	7	30
hamburger, kids' meal	1 meal	270	10	15	33	7	30
pita, chicken caesar	1 sandwich	480	19	30	48	5	60
pita, classic Greek	1 sandwich	440	20	16	50	6	25
pita, garden ranch chicken	1 sandwich	480	20	27	51	7	65
pita, garden veggie	1 sandwich	400	17	11	52	8	15
salad, caesar	1 salad	110	6	9	6	1	15
salad, grilled chicken	1 salad	190	8	22	10	5	45
salad, taco	1 salad	380	19	26	28	8	65
WHITE CASTLE							
breakfast sandwich	1 sandwich	340	25	14	17	2	130
cheeseburger	1 sandwich	235	14	7	11	0	20
cheeseburger, bacon	1 sandwich	200	13	10	12	0	25

Food	Portion	Calories	Fat	Protein	Carb	Sugar	Chol
cheeseburger, double	1 sandwich	285	18	14	12	0	30
cheese sticks	5 pieces	491	28	25	32		
chicken rings	6 pieces	310	21	16	17	2	70
chicken ring sandwich	1 sandwich	170	7	5	5		24
fish sandwich	1 sandwich	160	6	8	18	1	15
french fries	small	115	6		15	2	
hamburger	1 sandwich	135	7	6	11	0	10
hamburger, double	1 sandwich	235	14	11	16	0	20
onion rings	8 pieces	460	27	12	56		
shake, chocolate	14 oz	220	7	8	32	27	25
shake, vanilla	14 oz	230	7	8	35	28	25

FISH AND SEAFOOD

Food	Portion	Calories	Fat	Protein	Carb	Sugar	Chol
abalone, fried	3 oz	161	5.8	16.7	9.4		80
anchovy, canned in olive oil	5	42	1.9	5.8	0.0		17
anchovy paste	1 t	14	0.8	1.4	0.3		
bass, black, baked	3 oz	259	15.8	16.2	11.4		
bass, freshwater, cooked	3 oz	97	3.1	20.6	0.0		58
bass, striped, baked	3 oz	105	2.5	19.3	0.0		88
bluefish, baked	3 oz	135	4.6	21.8	0.0		65
catfish, baked	3 oz	129	6.8	15.9	0.0		54
catfish, breaded, fried	3 oz	195	11.3	15.4	6.8		69
catfish, frozen fillets	3 oz	210	12.6	15.7	19.2		42
caviar, black/red	1 T	40	2.9	3.9	0.6		94
clams, breaded, fried	3 oz	172	9.5	12.1	8.8		52
clams, raw	3 oz	63	0.8	10.9	2.2		29
clams, steamed	3 oz	126	1.7	21.7	4.4		57
cod, baked	3 oz	89	0.7	19.4	0.0		47
cod, dried/salted	3 oz	247	2.0	53.4	0.0		29

Food	Portion	Calories	Fat	Protein	Carb	Sugar	Chol
cod, frozen fillets	3 oz	177	7.4	15.3	26.5		28
crab, Alaska king, steamed	3 oz	82	1.3	16.5	0.0		45
crab, imitation (surimi)	3 oz	87	1.1	10.2	8.7		17
crab, blue, steamed	3 oz	87	1.5	17.2	0.0		85
crab cake	1 cake	93	4.5	12.1	0.3		90
crayfish, steamed	3 oz	74	1.1	14.9	0.0		117
fish cakes, frozen	3 oz	181	7.7	11.0	25.9		
fish fillets, frozen, in batter	3 oz	223	12.9	15.9	37.6		26
fish sticks, frozen	1 stick	77	3.5	4.4	6.7		32
flounder/sole, baked	3 oz	100	1.3	20.5	0.0		58
flounder/sole, breaded, frozen	3 oz	208	11.2	11.6	24.3		24
gefilte fish	1 piece	35	0.7	3.8	3.1		13
grouper, baked	3 oz	100	1.1	21.2	0.0		40
haddock, baked	3 oz	95	0.8	20.6	0.0		63
haddock, breaded, frozen	4 oz	316	16.0	11.3	31.4		
halibut, baked	3 oz	119	2.5	22.7			35
herring, pickled	1 piece	39	2.7	2.1	1.4		2
lobster, steamed	3 oz	83	0.5	17.4	1.1		61
mackerel, baked	3 oz	223	15.1	20.3	0.0		64
mackerel, jack, canned	1 cup	296	12.0	44.1	0.0		150
monkfish, baked	3 oz	82	1.7	15.8	0.0		27
mullet, baked	3 oz	128	4.1	21.1	0.0		54
mussels, steamed	3 oz	146	3.8	20.2	6.3		48
ocean perch, baked	3 oz	103	1.8	20.3	0.0		46
orange roughy, baked	3 oz	76	0.8	16.0	0.0		22
oysters, breaded, fried	3 oz	168	10.7	7.5	9.9		69
oysters, canned	3 oz	59	2.1	6.0	3.3		47

Food	Portion	Calories	Fat	Protein	Carb	Sugar	Chol
oysters, raw	6	50	1.3	4.4	4.6		21
perch, baked	3 oz	100	1.0	21.1	0.0		98
perch, breaded, frozen	3 oz	236	14.4	13.1	22.6		39
pike, baked	3 oz	96	0.7	21.0	0.0		43
pollock, baked	3 oz	100	1.1	21.2	0.0		77
pompano, baked	3 oz	179	10.3	20.1	0.0		54
sablefish, smoked	3 oz	219	17.1	15.0	0.0		54
salmon, Atlantic, baked	3 oz	175	10.5	18.8	0.0		54
salmon, smoked	3 oz	100	3.7	15.5	0.0		20
salmon, pink, canned	3 oz	118	5.1	16.8	0.0		47
salmon, sockeye, baked	3 oz	184	9.3	23.2	0.0		74
salmon, sockeye, canned	3 oz	130	6.2	17.4			37
sardines, canned in soybean oil	2 oz	50	2.7	5.9	0.0		34
scallops, breaded, fried	3 oz	67	3.4	5.6	3.1		19
sea bass, baked	3 oz	105	2.2	20.1	0.0		45
seatrout, baked	3 oz	88	3.1	18.3	0.0		71
shad, baked	3 oz	214	15.0	18.5	0.0		82
shrimp, breaded, fried	3 oz	206	10.4	18.2	9.8		151
shrimp, steamed	3 oz	84	0.9	17.8	0.0		166
snapper, baked	3 oz	109	1.5	22.4	0.0		40
squid, fried	3 oz	149	6.4	15.3	6.6		221
sturgeon, baked	3 oz	115	4.4	17.6	0.0		65
sturgeon, smoked	3 oz	147	3.7	26.5	0.0		68
surimi	3 oz	84	0.8	12.9	5.8		26
swordfish, baked	3 oz	132	4.4	21.6	0.0		43
tilefish, baked	3 oz	125	4.0	20.8	0.0		54
trout, rainbow, baked	3 oz	144	6.1	20.6	0.0		58
tuna, bluefin, baked	3 oz	156	5.3	25.4	0.0		42

Food	Portion	Calories	Fat	Protein	Carb	Sugar	Chol
tuna, light, canned in oil	3 oz	168	7.0	24.8	0.0		15
tuna, white, canned in oil	3 oz	158	6.9	22.6	0.0		26
tuna, light, canned in water	3 oz	99	0.7	21.7	0.0		26
tuna, white, canned in water	3 oz	109	2.5	20.1	0.0		36
turbot, baked	3 oz	104	3.2	17.5	0.0		53
whitefish, smoked	3 oz	92	0.8	19.9	0.0		28
whiting, baked	3 oz	77	1.1	15.6	0.0		57
yellowtail, baked	3 oz	124	4.5	19.7	0.0		47
FROZEN DINNERS							
beef, broccoli, Hunan, Lean Cuisine	1 meal	240	3.5	11.0	40.0	9.0	20
beef, chopped, Swanson Hungry Man	1 meal	602	30.2	38.4	44.1		
beef, roast, noodles, Budget Gourmet	1 meal	318	11.8	14.1	40.0		47
beef, sliced, Banquet	1 meal	240	7.0	26.0	19.0	12.0	70
beef, sliced, Swanson Hungry Man	1 meal	454	11.3	37.8	50.0		
beef, stroganoff, Healthy Choice	1 meal	310	6.0	21.0	44.0	19.0	60
beef tips, Healthy Choice	1 meal	260	6.0	20.0	32.0	18.0	40
chicken, a la king, Le Menu	1 meal	307	11.2	23.1	28.1		
chicken, alfredo, Green Giant	1 cup	270	6.0	19.0	35.0	5.0	35
chicken, baked, potatoes, Stouffer's	1 meal	330	14.0	25.0	25.0		60

Food	Portion	Calories	Fat	Protein	Carb	Sugar	Chol
chicken, BBQ meal, Tyson	1 meal	266	5.4	18.3	49.0	17.2	29
chicken, bowtie pasta, Lean Cuisine	1 meal	220	4.0	15.0	32.0	6.0	40
chicken, boneless, Swanson Hungry Man	1 meal	668	25.6	44.0	65.0		
chicken, broccoli alfredo, Healthy Choice	1 meal	300	6.0	25.0	38.0		40
chicken, cacciatore, Healthy Choice	1 meal	250	2.5	21.0	36.0	4.0	25
chicken, Cantonese, Healthy Choice	1 meal	260	2.0	25.0	35.0	6.0	40
chicken, cheese lasagna, Lean Cuisine	1 meal	270	8.0	16.0	34.0	6.0	35
chicken, cheesy pasta, Green Giant	1 cup	270	6.0	18.0	37.0	7.0	40
chicken, cordon bleu, Le Menu	1 meal	458	19.5	23.3	47.5		
chicken, dijon, Healthy Choice	1 meal	270	5.0	23.0	33.0	6.0	40
chicken, francesca, Healthy Choice	1 meal	330	6.0	23.0	46.0	0.0	30
chicken, fried, Banquet	1 meal	470	27.0	21.0	35.0	1.0	105
chicken, fried, Morton	1 meal	420	25.0	20.0	30.0	4.0	85
chicken, fried, Stouffer's	1 meal	310	12.0	17.0	33.0		45
chicken, fried, Swanson	1 meal	549	24.3	22.5	60.1		
chicken, garden herb, Birdseye	1 cup	310	15.0	16.0	28.0	8.0	40

Food	Portion	Calories	Fat	Protein	Carb	Sugar	Chol
chicken, garlic pasta, Green Giant	1 cup	250	7.0	16.0	30.0	3.0	40
chicken, roasted, Marie Callender	1 meal	670	42.0	43.0	32.0		205
chicken, kiev, Tyson	1 meal	443	25.0	17.7	36.4	3.9	84
chicken, mandarin, Budget Gourmet	1 meal	240	6.0	8.0	35.0		20
chicken, marsala, Tyson	1 meal	180	5.0	14.9	18.8	6.3	29
chicken, mesquite, Tyson	1 meal	308	7.1	22.9	38.1	13.3	40
chicken nuggets, Banquet	1 meal	410	21.0	18.0	38.0	11.0	45
chicken nuggets, Morton	1 meal	320	17.0	13.0	30.0	12.0	30
chicken nuggets, Swanson Hungry Man	1 meal	596	25.5	23.4	68.4		
chicken, oriental, Le Menu	1 meal	321	7.6	21.6	41.8		
chicken, parmagiana, Banquet	1 meal	290	15.0	14.0	27.0	3.0	50
chicken, parmagiana, Healthy Choice	1 meal	300	4.0	20.0	47.0	13.0	35
chicken, parmagiana, Le Menu	1 meal	397	19.2	26.3	29.6		
chicken, roasted, Healthy Choice	1 meal	220	3.0	23.0	27.0	9.0	35
chicken, sweet and sour, Green Giant	1 cup	320	1.5	14.0	62.0	22.0	25
chicken, sweet and sour, Healthy Choice	1 meal	330	5.0	20.0	53.0	30.0	45

Food	Portion	Calories	Fat	Protein	Carb	Sugar	Chol
chicken, sweet and sour, Swanson	1 meal	381	11.6	21.4	47.4		
chicken, teriyaki, Green Giant	1 cup	250	1.5	15.0	45.0	8.0	25
chicken, teriyaki, Healthy Choice	1 meal	230	3.0	19.0	32.0	8.0	45
chicken, vegetables, Lean Cuisine	1 meal	250	5.0	18.0	33.0	4.0	30
chimichanga, Banquet	1 meal	470	23.0	13.0	56.0	9.0	15
enchilada, beef, Banquet	1 meal	380	12.0	15.0	54.0	7.0	15
enchilada, beef, Patio	1 meal	350	10.0	12.0	52.0	2.0	15
enchilada, beef, Swanson	1 meal	475	20.5	17.2	55.4		
enchilada, cheese, Banquet	1 meal	340	6.0	15.0	56.0	7.0	15
enchilada, cheese, Patio	1 meal	330	8.0	13.0	52.0	7.0	15
enchilada, chicken, Banquet	1 meal	360	10.0	15.0	54.0	7.0	20
fish 'n chips, Swanson	1 meal	497	19.8	19.8	59.9		
fish, herb baked, Healthy Choice	1 meal	340	7.0				35
fish, lemon pepper, Healthy Choice	1 meal	290	5.0	14.0	47.0	20.0	25
fish, macaroni and cheese, Stouffer's	1 meal	460	20.0	22.0	47.0		55
lasagna, meat sauce, Banquet	1 meal	260	8.0	12.0	35.0	10.0	10
macaroni and cheese, Banquet	1 meal	320	11.0	12.0	43.0	6.0	20
macaroni and cheese, Swanson	1 meal	373	14.4	12.9	47.9		

Food	Portion	Calories	Fat	Protein	Carb	Sugar	Chol
meatloaf, Banquet	1 meal	280	16.0	13.0	22.0	3.0	80
meatloaf, Healthy Choice	1 meal	320	5.0	15.0	52.0	17.0	35
meatloaf, Lean Cuisine	1 meal	260	7.0	20.0	28.0	5.0	45
pepper steak, Le Menu	1 meal	354	12.5	25.8	34.7		
pork chop, fried, Marie Callender	1 meal	550	27.0	26.0	50.0	16.0	65
pork loin, Swanson	1 meal	282	10.6	20.4	26.2		
pot roast, Healthy Choice	1 meal	280	5.0	19.0	38.0	20.0	45
pot roast, Le Menu	1 meal	316	12.0	25.6	26.5		
pot roast, noodles, Marie Callender	1 meal	500	17.0	23.0	55.0		110
pot roast, potatoes, Stouffer's	1 meal	250	8.0	16.0	29.0		35
pot roast, Swanson	1 meal	406	10.4	30.1	48.0		
Salisbury steak, Banquet	1 meal	340	19.0	15.0	28.0	4.0	60
Salisbury steak, Healthy Choice	1 meal	320	6.0	18.0	48.0	20.0	45
Salisbury steak, Morton	1 meal	210	9.0	9.0	23.0	7.0	20
Salisbury steak, Swanson	1 meal	409	17.9	18.9	43.2		
shrimp, angel hair pasta, Lean Cuisine	1 meal	280	5.0	15.0	44.0	7.0	60
sirloin, chopped, Swanson	1 meal	356	17.8	21.1	27.9		
sirloin steak, potatoes, Birdseye	1 cup	240	9.0	13.0	26.0	5.0	25
sirloin tips, Le Menu	1 meal	383	17.5	29.5	26.7		

Food	Portion	Calories	Fat	Protein	Carb	Sugar	Chol
tamales, beef, Swanson	1 meal	352	12.9	13.4	45.5		
tamales, chicken, Swanson	1 meal	325	12.5	7.9	45.2		
turkey, Banquet	1 meal	270	12.0	11.0	29.0		30
turkey, Stouffer's	1 meal	320	13.0	19.0	31.0		50
turkey, Swanson	1 meal	350	11.1	20.1	42.5		
turkey, Swanson Hungry Man	1 meal	537	16.1	36.3	61.8		
turkey, potatoes, Birdseye	1 cup	200	6.0	12.0	24.0	4.0	10
turkey, white meat, Banquet	1 meal	290	10.0	17.0	34.0	7.0	55
turkey, white meat, Le Menu	1 meal	325	13.0	28.0	24.0		
turkey, white meat, Marie Callender	1 meal	310	10.0	22.0	34.0		40
veal, marsala, Le Menu	1 meal	250	5.2	25.3	25.4	0.0	112
veal, parmagiana, vegetables, Banquet	1 meal	360	19.0	13.0	35.0		25
veal, parmagiana, Banquet	1 meal	320	14.0	13.0	35.0	4.0	25
veal, parmagiana, spaghetti, Stouffer's	1 meal	430	17.0	21.0	49.0		80
veal, parmagiana, Swanson	1 meal	441	20.3	21.9	42.7		
ziti, meat sauce, Swanson	1 meal	558	23.5	28.4	58.4		
FROZEN ENTREES beef, burgundy, Le Menu	1 entree	316	18.5	25.1	12.3		
beef, macaroni, Healthy Choice	1 entree	210	2.0	14.0	34.0	9.0	15

Food	Portion	Calories	Fat	Protein	Carb	Sugar	Chol
beef, oriental, Lean Cuisine	1 entree	270	8.0	20.0	30.0		45
beef, patties, Banquet	1 entree	180	14.0	8.0	7.0	5.0	20
beef, peppercorn, Lean Cuisine	1 entree	260	7.0	16.0	32.0	5.0	25
beef, portabello, Lean Cuisine	1 entree	220	7.0	14.0	24.0	6.0	35
beef, sliced, Banquet	1 entree	70	2.0				25
beef, stroganoff, Budget Gourmet	1 entree	250	7.0	16.0	30.0		35
beef, stroganoff, Stouffer's	1 entree	390	20.0	23.0	30.0		85
beef, szechuan, Lean Cuisine	1 entree	280	11.0	20.0	25.0		95
beef stew, Stouffer's	1 entree	129	6.8	9.7	7.2		28
beef tips, Southern, Lean Cuisine	1 entree	270	6.0	16.0	37.0	10.0	35
burrito, beef and bean, Patio	1 entree	280	7.0	10.0	45.0	5.0	15
burrito, beef and cheese, Patio	1 entree	270	5.0	9.0	46.0	2.0	5
burrito, chicken, Patio	1 entree	260	4.0	12.0	44.0	5.0	15
cabbage, stuffed, beef, Lean Cuisine	1 entree	210	8.0	9.0	25.0	4.0	20
cabbage, stuffed, beef, Stouffer's	1 entree	97	4.3	6.0	8.5		14
cannelloni, cheese, Stouffer's	1 entree	172	8.3	10.1	13.7		20
chicken, a la king, Le Menu	1 entree	241	5.0	17.9	31.0		29
chicken, a la king, Stouffer's	1 entree	350	13.0	17.0	41.0		40
chicken, a l'orange, Lean Cuisine	1 entree	230	1.5	20.0	33.0	9.0	40

Food	Portion	Calories	Fat	Protein	Carb	Sugar	Chol
chicken, baked, Lean Cuisine	1 entree	240	4.5	17.0	33.0	4.0	30
chicken, basil cream, Lean Cuisine	1 entree	290	7.0	19.0	37.0	3.0	35
chicken, BBQ glazed, Weight Watchers	1 entree	230	4.0	20.0	33.1		30
chicken, breast strips, Weaver	3 strips	210	11.0	14.0	13.0	1.0	35
chicken, cacciatore, Lean Cuisine	1 entree	280	10.0	23.0	25.0		45
chicken, carbonara, Lean Cuisine	1 entree	260	8.0	17.0	29.0	6.0	30
chicken, cordon bleu, Weight Watchers	1 entree	230	2.0	15.0	31.1		20
chicken, croquettes, Weaver	2 pieces	340	21.0	15.0	22.0	6.0	45
chicken, creamed, Stouffer's	1 entree	260	19.0	15.0	8.0		80
chicken, crispy mini-drums, Weaver	5 pieces	250	16.0	14.0	14.0	2.0	40
chicken, dijon, Le Menu	1 entree	229	6.6	20.5	22.1		36
chicken, dumplings, Banquet	1 entree	290	14.0	12.0	30.0	2.0	40
chicken, fettucine, Healthy Choice	1 entree	260	4.5	22.0	35.0	3.0	40
chicken, fried, Banquet	1 entree	272	18.1	14.1	13.1		65
chicken, fried, Marie Callender	1 entree	610	27.0	25.0	67.0		55
chicken, glazed, Healthy Choice	1 entree	210	2.0	17.0	31.0	1.0	30

Food	Portion	Calories	Fat	Protein	Carb	Sugar	Chol
chicken, glazed, Lean Cuisine	1 entree	270	8.0	26.0	23.0		60
chicken, grilled, Lean Cuisine	1 entree	260	4.5	15.0	40.0	4.0	35
chicken, herb roasted, Lean Cuisine	1 entree	200	3.5	17.0	24.0	5.0	35
chicken, herb sauce, Lean Cuisine	1 entree	260	10.0	23.0	19.0		80
chicken, honey mustard, Lean Cuisine	1 entree	270	3.5	19.0	40.0	8.0	35
chicken, kiev, Le Menu	1 entree	491	31.6	18.1	33.0		
chicken, mandarin, Budget Gourmet	1 entree	270	8.0	10.0	39.0		30
chicken, marsala, Healthy Choice	1 entree	230	1.5	25.0	11.0		30
chicken, marsala, Lean Cuisine	1 entree	190	5.0	25.0	11.0		75
chicken, Mediterranean, Lean Cuisine	1 entree	260	4.0	17.0	38.0	6.0	20
chicken, mexicali, Stouffer's	1 entree	119	4.9	8.3	10.7		29
chicken, noodles, Marie Callender	1 entree	271	16.0	10.0	22.1		20
chicken, noodles, Stouffer's	1 entree	254	12.5	18.2	17.5		54
chicken, nuggets, Weaver	1 entree	210	15.0	11.0	9.0	0.0	35
chicken, oriental, Lean Cuisine	1 entree	240	6.0	23.0	23.0		100
chicken, parmesan, Lean Cuisine	1 entree	250	8.0	25.0	19.0		70
chicken, parmigiana, Weight Watchers	1 entree	310	4.0	21.0	39.0		30

Food	Portion	Calories	Fat	Protein	Carb	Sugar	Chol
chicken, peanut sauce, Lean Cuisine	1 entree	260	6.0	20.0	32.0	7.0	30
chicken, piccata, Lean Cuisine	1 entree	300	9.0	14.0	41.0	9.0	30
chicken, primavera, Stouffer's	1 entree	66	2.3	6.7	4.6		17
chicken, rondelets, Weaver	1 piece	180	11.0	10.0	10.0	1.0	30
chicken, sesame	1 entree	240	3.0	16.0	38.0	9.0	30
chicken, sweet/ sour, Lean Cuisine	1 entree	320	3.0	17.0	57.0	18.0	30
chicken, tenders, Weaver	5 pieces	220	15.0	14.0	8.0	0.0	35
chicken, tenders, honey, Weaver	5 pieces	230	15.0	12.0	12.0	3.0	35
chicken, teriyaki, Lean Cuisine	1 entree	320	3.5	21.0	51.0	11.0	40
chicken, Thai-style, Lean Cuisine	1 entree	270	5.0	16.0	39.0	7.0	30
chicken, vegetables, Lean Cuisine	1 entree	270	7.0	23.0	29.0		45
chicken, wine sauce, Lean Cuisine	1 entree	220	5.0	20.0	23.0	7.0	45
chicken, wings, honey BBQ, Weaver	3 pieces	200	11.0	17.0	7.0	2.0	95
chili, beef, Stouffer's	1 entree	111	6.6	7.7	5.2		26
chili with beans, Stouffer's	1 entree	259	9.8	20.7	21.8		50
chow mein, chicken, Lean Cuisine	1 entree	250	5.0	14.0	36.0		30
eggplant parmigiana, Celentano	1 entree	350	28.0	9.0	17.0	6.0	70

Food	Portion	Calories	Fat	Protein	Carb	Sugar	Chol
egg rolls, chicken, Chun King	1 entree	170	5.0	7.0	25.0	4.0	10
egg rolls, chicken, La Choy	1 entree	170	5.0	7.0	25.0	4.0	10
egg rolls, pork, Chun King	1 entree	170	6.0	6.0	23.0	6.0	5
egg rolls, shrimp, Chun King	1 entree	150	4.0	6.0	24.0	6.0	10
enchilada, beef, Patio	1 entree	200	6.0	5.0	31.0	1.0	10
enchilada, cheese, Patio	1 entree	170	4.0	6.0	26.0	3.0	10
fajita, chicken, Healthy Choice	1 entree	260	4.0	21.0	36.0	6.0	30
fettucini alfredo, Healthy Choice	1 entree	250	5.0	11.0	39.0	4.0	15
fish, baked, Lean Cuisine	1 entree	290	6.0	20.0	40.0	6.0	40
fish, florentine, Lean Cuisine	1 entree	240	9.0	27.0	13.0		100
fish 'n chips, Swansons	1 entree	363	16.5	14.0	39.4		
lasagna, Banquet	1 entree	230	8.0	12.0	29.0	1.0	35
lasagna, Lean Cuisine	1 entree	280	8.0	27.0	24.0		70
lasagna, vegetable, Stouffer's	1 entree	338	16.6	19.3	28.1		39
lasagna, zucchini, Healthy Choice	1 entree	330	1.5	20.0	58.0	11.0	10
linguini, clam sauce, Lean Cuisine	1 entree	260	7.0	16.0	32.0		30
macaroni, beef, Stouffer's	1 entree	110	12.0	20.0	26.0		35
macaroni, beef, Swanson	1 entree	265	9.2	19.8	25.6		
macaroni and cheese, Banquet	1 entree	210	5.0	8.0	33.0	7.0	10

Food	Portion	Calories	Fat	Protein	Carb	Sugar	Chol
macaroni and cheese, Healthy Choice	1 entree	290	5.0	15.0	45.0	13.0	15
manicotti, 3 cheese, Healthy Choice	1 entree	260	4.5	16.0	40.0	7.0	25
meatballs, Italian, Celentano	1 entree	250	19.0	14.0	5.0	1.0	55
meatballs, Italian, Swanson	1 entree	483	15.9	24.5	60.4		
meatballs, Swedish, Healthy Choice	1 entree	280	9.0	22.0	35.0	4.0	60
meatloaf, Stouffer's	1 entree	360	20.0	20.0	26.0		
meatloaf with gravy, Banquet	1 entree	160	10.0	10.0	8.0	1.0	35
noodles romanoff, Stouffer's	1 entree	130	7.1	5.4	11.1		14
oriental beef, Budget Gourmet	1 entree	240	7.0	10.0	34.0		25
pasta roma, Stouffer's	1 entree	204	5.9	12.7	24.7		24
penne, pork/ tomato, Healthy Choice	1 entree	230	5.0	9.0	36.0	3.0	10
pepper steak, Healthy Choice	1 entree	250	4.0	19.0	34.0	0.0	35
pepper steak, Stouffer's	1 entree	330	9.0	17.0	45.0		35
pepper steak, Weight Watchers	1 entree	240	4.5	18.0	33.0		35
pork, honey roasted, Lean Cuisine	1 entree	240	5.0	17.0	31.0	10.0	45
pot pie, beef, Banquet	1 entree	330	15.0	9.0	38.0	2.0	25
pot pie, beef, Swanson	1 entree	364	19.0				

Food	Portion	Calories	Fat	Protein	Carb	Sugar	Chol
pot pie, beef, Swanson Chunky	1 entree	575	29.2	20.1	58.1		
pot pie, chicken, Banquet	1 entree	350	18.0	10.0	36.0	2.0	40
pot pie, chicken, Marie Callender	1 entree	619	31.0	13.0	48.9		15
pot pie, chicken, Stouffer's	1 entree	540	33.0	23.0	38.0		25
pot pie, chicken, Swanson	1 entree	379	21.7	11.1	34.9		
pot pie, chicken, Tyson	1 entree	567	36.6	13.6	45.8	2.1	23
pot pie, chicken, broccoli, Marie Callender	1 entree	799	48.9	20.0	60.9		20
pot pie, macaroni/ cheese, Banquet	1 entree	200	3.0	7.0	35.0	2.0	10
pot pie, turkey, Banquet	1 entree	371	20.1	10.0	38.1	3.0	45
pot pie, turkey/ vegetable, Morton	1 entree	311	17.0	7.0	34.1		15
pot pie, turkey, Stouffer's	1 entree	530	33.0	21.0	36.0		65
pot pie, turkey, Swanson	1 entree	381	21.4	10.9	36.1		
pot pie, turkey, Tyson	1 entree	552	32.9	14.9	49.2	5.7	22
pot pie, Yankee, Marie Callender	1 entree	641	39.0	19.0	53.0		10
pot roast, Lean Cuisine	1 entree	190	6.0	15.0	19.0	4.0	30
pot roast, Marie Callender	1 entree	250	6.0	17.0	31.0	5.0	45
ravioli, cheese, Healthy Choice	1 entree	260	5.0	11.0	44.0	14.0	20
ravioli, cheese, Swanson	1 entree	273	7.5	12.8	38.7		
rigatoni, meat sauce, Lean Cuisine	1 entree	260	10.0	18.0	25.0		35

Food	Portion	Calories	Fat	Protein	Carb	Sugar	Chol
salisbury steak, Banquet	1 entree	220	16.0	9.0	8.0	1.0	25
salisbury steak, Budget Gourmet	1 entree	240	7.0	16.0	27.0		10
salisbury steak, Morton's	1 entree	210	9.0	9.0	23.0		20
salisbury steak, Stouffer's	1 entree	241	14.6	17.0	10.2		73
salisbury steak, Weight Watchers	1 entree	150	9.0	19.0	24.0		40
shells, cheese-stuffed, Stouffer's	1 entree	268	8.5	14.9	33.3		24
shrimp, marinara, Weight Watchers	1 entree	200	2.0	8.0	37.1		40
sirloin tips, noodles, Stouffer's	1 entree	258	10.2	18.9	22.6		
spaghetti, beef sauce, Healthy Choice	1 entree	260	3.0	14.0	43.0	7.0	15
spaghetti, meat sauce, Marie Callender	1 entree	260	10.0	11.0	32.0	5.0	5
stuffed pepper, beef, Stouffer's	1 entree	192	8.6	10.2	18.6		22
Swedish meatballs, Celentano	6 meatballs	260	19.0	12.0	5.0	1.0	45
Swedish meatballs, Lean Cuisine	1 entree	290	7.0	22.0	35.0	4.0	45
Swedish meatballs, Weight Watchers	1 entree	290	7.0	18.0	34.0		30
tortellini, beef, Stouffer's	1 entree	238	8.3	15.4	25.6		83
tortellini, cheese, Stouffer's	1 entree	268	10.9	15.4	26.9		77
tortellini, chicken, Stouffer's	1 entree	241	7.4	15.4	28.2		81
tuna noodle casserole, Stouffer's	1 entree	320	10.0	20.0	37.0		40

Food	Portion	Calories	Fat	Protein	Carb	Sugar	Chol
tuna noodle casserole, Swanson	1 entree	259	7.9	13.4	33.5		
turkey, dijon, Lean Cuisine	1 entree	280	10.0	26.0	21.0		65
turkey, gravy, Banquet	1 entree	140	9.0	8.0	6.0	0.0	30
turkey, dressing, Marie Callender	1 entree	530	17.0	33.0	51.0		85
turkey, glazed, Lean Cuisine	1 entree	260	4.5	14.0	41.0	20.0	25
turkey, stuffed breast, Weight Watchers	1 entree	230	6.0	17.0	28.1		15
turkey, tetrazzini, Stouffer's	1 entree	360	17.0	19.0	33.0		55
veal, parmagiana, Le Menu	1 entree	174	5.5	21.9	9.0		97
veal, parmagiana, Morton	1 entree	280	13.0	8.0	30.0		20
FRUIT							
apple, raw	1 medium	81	0.5	0.3	21.0	18.4	0
applesauce, sweetened	½ cup	97	0.2	0.2	25.5	21.1	0
apricots, canned, syrup	4 halves	75	0.1	0.5	19.3		0
apricots, raw	3 medium	106	0.4	1.5	11.8	9.0	0
avocado, California, raw	1 medium	306	30.0	3.7	12.0		0
avocado, Florida, raw	1 medium	340	27.0	4.8	27.1		0
banana, raw	1 medium	105	0.5	1.2	26.7	17.8	0
blackberries, frozen, unsweetened	1 cup	97	0.6	1.8	23.7		0
blackberries, raw	½ cup	37	0.3	0.5	9.2		0
blueberries, frozen, sweetened	1 cup	186	0.3	0.9	50.5		0

Food	Portion	Calories	Fat	Protein	Carb	Sugar	Chol
blueberries, raw	1 cup	81	0.6	1.0	20.5	10.6	0
cantaloupe, raw	1 cup	56	0.4	1.4	13.4	3.9	0
casaba melon, raw	1 cup	44	0.2	1.5	10.5		0
cherries, sour, canned, syrup	½ cup	116	0.1	0.9	29.8		0
cherries, sweet, frozen, sweetened	1 cup	231	0.3	3.0	57.9		0
cherries, sweet, raw	10 cherries	49	0.7	0.8	11.3		0
cranberries, raw	1 cup	47	0.2	0.4	12.0		0
cranberry sauce, jellied	½ cup	208	0.2	0.3	53.7		0
dates, dried	10 dates	228	0.4	1.6	61.0	53.3	0
figs, canned, syrup	3 figs	75	0.1	0.3	19.5		0
figs, dried	10 figs	477	2.2	5.7	122.2		0
figs, raw	1 medium	37	0.1	0.4	9.6		0
fruit cocktail, canned, heavy syrup	½ cup	93	0.1	0.5	24.2		0
fruit salad, canned, heavy syrup	½ cup	93	0.1	0.4	24.5		0
grapefruit, canned, heavy syrup	½ cup	76	0.1	0.7	19.6		0
grapefruit, raw, pink/red/white	½ medium	39	0.1	0.8	9.9		0
grapes, green/red	1 cup	58	0.3	0.6	15.8	15.1	0
guava, raw	1 medium	46	0.5	0.7	10.7		0
honeydew melon, raw	1 cup	60	0.2	0.8	15.6		0
kiwifruit, raw	1 medium	46	0.3	0.8	11.5	8.0	0
lemon, raw	1 medium	17	0.2	0.6	5.4	1.4	0
lime, raw	1 medium	20	0.1	0.5	7.1	0.3	0
mandarin oranges, canned, syrup	½ cup	77	0.1	0.6	20.4		0
mango, raw	1 medium	135	0.6	1.1	35.2		0

Food	Portion	Calories	Fat	Protein	Carb	Sugar	Chol
nectarine, raw	1 medium	67	0.6	1.3	16.0	12.1	0
orange, navel, raw	1 medium	60	0.1	1.3	15.2		0
papaya, raw	1 medium	119	0.4	1.9	29.8		0
passion fruit, raw	1 medium	17	0.1	0.4	4.2		0
peach, canned, heavy syrup	1 cup	189	0.3	1.2	51.0		0
peach, raw	1 medium	37	0.1	0.6	9.7	7.6	0
pear, canned, heavy syrup	1 cup	189	0.3	0.5	48.9	38.8	0
pear, raw	1 medium	98	0.7	0.6	25.1	17.4	0
persimmon, raw	1 medium	32	0.1	0.2	8.4		0
pineapple, canned, heavy syrup	1 cup	199	0.3	0.9	51.5		0
pineapple, raw	1 cup	76	0.7	0.6	19.2	18.4	0
plums, canned, heavy syrup	3 plums	118	0.1	0.5	30.9		0
plums, raw	1 medium	36	0.4	0.5	8.6	5.0	0
pomegranate, raw	1 medium	105	0.5	1.5	26.4		0
prunes, canned, heavy syrup	5 prunes	90	0.2	0.7	23.9		0
prunes, dried	10 prunes	201	0.4	2.2	52.7		0
raisins, golden	⅔ cup	302	0.5	3.4	79.5		0
raisins, dark	⅔ cup	296	0.5	2.5	78.5		0
raspberries, frozen, sweetened	⅔ cup	103	0.2	0.7	26.2		0
raspberries, raw	1 cup	60	0.7	1.1	14.2		0
strawberries, frozen, sweetened	1 cup	199	0.4	1.3	53.5		0
strawberries, raw	1 cup	45	0.6	0.9	10.5	8.6	0
tangerine, raw	1 medium	37	0.2	0.5	9.4		0
watermelon, raw	1 cup	51	0.7	1.0	11.5		0

GELATIN, PUDDING, FROZEN DESSERTS

custard, baked	½ cup	209	6.6	7.2	15.1		123
custard, from mix	½ cup	162	5.5	5.5	23.4		81
flan, from mix	½ cup	150	4.1	4.0	25.4		16

Food	Portion	Calories	Fat	Protein	Carb	Sugar	Chol
gelatin from mix, all flavors	½ cup	83	0.0	1.7	19.6		0
gelatin, all flavors, Jell-O	½ cup	80	0.0	2.0	19.0	19.0	0
Gelatin Snacks, Jell-O	3.5 oz	80	0.0	1.0	18.0	18.0	0
ice cream, butter pecan	½ cup	236	13.9	4.2	23.8		
ice cream, chocolate	½ cup	143	7.3	2.5	18.6		22
ice cream, strawberry	½ cup	127	5.5	2.1	18.2		19
ice cream, vanilla	½ cup	133	7.3	2.3	15.6		29
ice cream bar, chocolate	1 bar	361	24.7	4.9	29.4		
ice cream bar, vanilla	1 bar	332	22.6	4.5	27.4		
ice pop	1 bar	42	0.0	0.0	11.2		0
mousse, chocolate	½ cup	446	33.0	8.7	33.0		299
pudding, banana, from mix	½ cup	157	4.2	4.1	25.3		17
pudding, banana, packaged	3.5 oz	119	4.5	1.5	18.3	13.8	2
pudding, bread	½ cup	212	7.4	6.6	31.0		83
pudding, butterscotch, packaged	3.5 oz	130	4.4	1.5	21.2	13.7	2
pudding, chocolate, instant mix	½ cup	158	4.4	4.4	26.7		16
pudding, chocolate, packaged	3.5 oz	143	5.4	2.0	21.7	17.4	1
pudding, lemon, cook and serve, Jell-O	½ cup	140	2.0	1.0	29.0	23.0	75
pudding, lemon, from mix	½ cup	169	4.3	4.0	29.5		16
pudding, rice	½ cup	152	4.3	5.5	40.1		17

Food	Portion	Calories	Fat	Protein	Carb	Sugar	Chol
pudding, rice, from mix	½ cup	176	4.0	4.8	30.0		16
pudding, tapioca	½ cup	190	6.5	7.1	25.8		15
pudding, tapioca, from mix	½ cup	161	4.1	4.1	27.6		17
pudding, vanilla	½ cup	130	4.1	4.1	19.6		16
pudding, vanilla, from mix	½ cup	155	4.2	4.1	25.9		17
puddings, cook and serve, Jell-O	½ cup	148	2.8	4.3	27.0	21.9	10
puddings, instant mix, Jell-O	½ cup	155	2.9	4.0	29.4	24.0	10
Pudding Snacks, Jell-O	4 oz	159	5.1	2.76	26.3	21.6	0
sherbet, orange	½ cup	132	1.9	1.1	29.2		5
yogurt, frozen	½ cup	115	4.3	2.9	17.9		4

MEATS
BEEF

Food	Portion	Calories	Fat	Protein	Carb	Sugar	Chol
brisket, braised	3.5 oz	291	19.5	26.8			93
chuck roast	3.5 oz	363	27.8	26.2			103
corned beef	3.5 oz	251	19.0	18.2	0.5		98
flank steak, braised	3.5 oz	263	16.4	27.0			72
ground, extra lean, broiled	3.5 oz	256	16.3	25.4			84
ground, lean, broiled	3.5 oz	272	18.5	24.7			87
ground, regular, broiled	3.5 oz	289	20.7	24.1			90
liver, braised	3.5 oz	161	4.9	24.4	3.4		389
pot roast, chuck	3.5 oz	348	25.8	27.0			99
prime ribs, roasted	3.5 oz	402	33.9	22.5			85
short ribs, braised	3.5 oz	471	42.0	21.6			94
round, bottom, roasted	3.5 oz	260	16.4	26.4			80

Food	Portion	Calories	Fat	Protein	Carb	Sugar	Chol
round, eye of, roasted	3.5 oz	241	14.1	26.6			72
round, top, broiled	3.5 oz	215	8.9	31.7			84
steak, porterhouse	3.5 oz	327	25.6	22.4			75
steak, sirloin	3.5 oz	229	11.6	29.2			89
steak, T-bone	3.5 oz	309	23.3	23.2			67
steak, tenderloin	3.5 oz	304	21.8	25.1			86
LAMB							
ground, broiled	3.5 oz	283	19.6	24.8			97
chop, loin	3.5 oz	316	23.1	25.2			100
chop, rib	3.5 oz	361	29.6	22.1			99
chop, shoulder	3.5 oz	281	19.6	24.4			96
leg, roasted	3.5 oz	225	12.4	26.4			90
stew pieces	3.5 oz	223	8.8	33.7			108
LUNCHEON MEATS							
bologna, beef	1 slice	72	6.6	2.8	0.2	0.5	13
bologna, beef, Boar's Head	2 oz	150	13.0	7.0	0.0	0.0	35
bologna, beef and pork	1 slice	73	6.5	2.7	0.6		13
bologna, beef and pork, Boar's Head	2 oz	150	13.0	7.0	1.0	0.0	35
bratwurst, Boar's Head	1 wurst	300	25.0	19.0	0.0	0.0	75
braunschweiger	1 slice	65	5.8	2.4	0.6		28
chicken breast, baked	2 slices	44	0.3	8.8	1.7	0.3	23
chicken breast, roasted, Boar's Head	2 oz	50	1.0	11.0	1.0	0.0	30
corned beef, Boar's Head	2 oz	80	3.5	12.0	0.0	0.0	40
frankfurter, beef	1 frank	180	16.2	6.8	1.0		35
frankfurter, beef, Boar's Head	1 frank	160	14.0	7.0	1.0	0.0	30

Food	Portion	Calories	Fat	Protein	Carb	Sugar	Chol
frankfurter, beef and pork	1 frank	182	16.6	6.4	1.5	1.1	28
frankfurter, turkey	1 frank	102	8.0	6.4	0.7		48
ham, baked	2 slices	47	1.2	8.0	1.0	1.0	24
ham, Black Forest, Boar's Head	2 oz	60	1.0	10.0	2.0	2.0	30
ham, cappy, Boar's Head	2 oz	60	1.5	10.0	3.0	2.0	15
ham, maple-glazed, Boar's Head	2 oz	60	1.0	10.0	3.0	3.0	20
ham, smoked, Boar's Head	2 oz	60	1.0	9.0	2.0	2.0	25
ham, spiced, Boar's Head	2 oz	120	10.0	7.0	1.0	0.0	30
head cheese, Boar's Head	2 oz	90	5.0	10.0	1.0	0.0	65
kielbasa, Boar's Head	2 oz	120	10.0	9.0	0.0	0.0	50
knockwurst, beef, Boar's Head	1 wurst	310	27.0	15.0	1.0	0.0	50
liverwurst, Boar's Head	2 oz	170	15.0	8.0	1.0	1.0	85
mortadella	1 slice	47	3.8	2.5	0.5		8
olive loaf	1 slice	66	4.6	3.3	2.6		11
olive loaf, Boar's Head	2 oz	130	12.0	6.0	1.0	0.0	20
pastrami, Boar's Head	2 oz	90	4.0	12.0	2.0	0.0	30
pastrami, turkey, Boar's Head	2 oz	60	0.5	13.0	1.0	0.0	25
prosciutto, Boar's Head	1 oz	60	3.0	8.0	0.0	0.0	15
roast beef, Boar's Head	2 oz	80	2.0	14.0	0.0	0.0	35
roast beef, Italian-style, Boar's Head	2 oz	80	2.0	12.0	2.0	0.0	40

Food	Portion	Calories	Fat	Protein	Carb	Sugar	Chol
salami, beef	1 slice	60	4.8	3.5	0.6		15
salami, beef, Boar's Head	2 oz	120	9.0	10.0	0.0	0.0	35
salami, cooked, Boar's Head	2 oz	130	11.0	8.0	0.0	0.0	40
salami, Genoa, Boar's Head	2 oz	180	14.0	12.0	1.0	0.0	55
salami, cotto	2 slices	93	7.1	6.5	0.9	0.5	38
salami, hard	1 slice	41	3.4	2.3	0.2		8
salami, hard, Boar's Head	1 oz	110	9.0	6.0	1.0	0.0	25
smoked link sausage, beef	1 link	128	11.5	5.4	0.8	0.5	27
smoked link sausage, pork	1 link	265	21.6	15.1	1.4		46
turkey breast	1 slice	23	0.3	4.7			9
turkey breast, smoked, Boar's Head	2 oz	60	0.5	13.0	0.0	0.0	30
vienna sausage	1 sausage	45	4.0	1.6	0.3		8
PORK							
bacon	2 slices	70	5.8	4.4	0.1	0.1	15
bacon, Canadian style	2 slices	87	4.0	11.4			27
chop, center rib, broiled	3.5 oz	260	15.8	27.6			82
chop, loin, broiled	3.5 oz	240	13.1	28.7			82
ham, cooked canned	3.5 oz	190	13.0	17.0			39
loin roast	3.5 oz	240	13.1	28.7			82
picnic, roasted	3.5 oz	280	21.4	20.4			58
sausage, fresh	1 link	48	4.1	2.6	0.1	0.3	11
spareribs, braised	3.5 oz	296	21.5	23.9			87
VEAL							
chop, loin, braised	3.5 oz	284	17.2	30.2			118
ground, broiled	3.5 oz	172	7.6	24.4			103

Food	Portion	Calories	Fat	Protein	Carb	Sugar	Chol
liver, braised	3.5 oz	165	6.9	21.6			561
rib, roasted	3.5 oz	251	12.5	24.0			139
stew, braised	3.5 oz	188	4.3	34.9			145

MILK AND YOGURT
MILK

Food	Portion	Calories	Fat	Protein	Carb	Sugar	Chol
buttermilk, cultured	8 oz	99	2.2	8.1	11.7	11.8	9
chocolate, whole	8 oz	208	8.5	7.9	25.9		31
cocoa, from mix	6 oz	103	1.2	3.1	22.5		2
condensed, sweetened	1 oz	122	3.3	3.0	20.7		13
eggnog, no alcohol	8 oz	342	19.0	9.7	34.4	·	149
evaporated, canned	1 oz	43	2.4	2.2	3.2		9
lowfat, 1%	8 oz	102	2.6	8.0	11.7		10
lowfat, 2%	8 oz	122	4.7	8.1	11.7		18
malted milk	8 oz	236	9.8	10.3	27.3		37
nonfat	8 oz	86	0.4	8.4	11.9	10.8	4
soy milk	8 oz	79	4.6	6.6	4.3		0
whole	8 oz	157	8.9	8.0	11.3		35

MILK AND SHAKE MIXES

Food	Portion	Calories	Fat	Protein	Carb	Sugar	Chol
Alba chocolate	1 packet	70	1.0	6.0	11.0		
Alba vanilla	1 packet	70	0.0	5.0	12.0		
chocolate milk powder, Hershey	3 T	111	0.3	0.5	22.3	20.9	0
cocoa mix, Swiss Miss	1 packet	110	1.8	1.7	22.6	20.7	1
Instant Breakfast, Carnation, chocolate	8 oz	130	1.5	4.5	26.0	17.0	3
Instant Breakfast, Carnation, strawberry	8 oz	130	0.2	5.4	26.4		

Food	Portion	Calories	Fat	Protein	Carb	Sugar	Chol
Instant Breakfast, Pillsbury, chocolate	8 oz	130	0.5	5.7	25.7		
Instant Breakfast, Pillsbury, vanilla	8 oz	133	0.2	5.4	27.3		
Weight Watchers, chocolate fudge	1 packet	79	1.0	5.9	11.8		0
YOGURT							
low fat, plain	8 oz	130	3.0	11.0	15.0	15.0	20
nonfat, plain	8 oz	130	0.0	13.0	19.0	14.0	10
whole, plain	8 oz	139	7.4	7.9	10.6		29
NUTS AND SEEDS							
almonds, dry roasted	1 oz	166	14.6	4.6	6.9	1.7	0
almonds, honey roasted	1 oz	169	14.1	5.2	7.9		0
almonds, oil roasted	1 oz	173	16.1	5.7	4.4		0
cashew butter	1 oz	16	14.0	5.0	7.8		0
cashews, dry roasted	1 oz	163	13.1	4.3	9.3		0
cashews, honey roasted	1 oz	150	13.0	4.0	7.0		0
cashews, oil roasted	1 oz	163	13.7	5.0	8.0		0
chestnuts, roasted	1 oz	69	0.6	0.9	15.0		0
coconut, dried, sweetened, flaked	1 cup	361	23.8	2.4	35.2		0
hazelnuts (filberts), dry roasted	1 oz	188	18.8	2.8	5.1		0
macadamia nuts, dry roasted	1 oz	200	21.1	2.5	3.2		0
mixed nuts, dry roasted	1 oz	168	14.6	4.9	7.2		0

Food	Portion	Calories	Fat	Protein	Carb	Sugar	Chol
peanut butter, chunky	2 T	188	16.0	7.7	6.9	3.5	0
peanut butter, smooth	2 T	190	16.3	8.1	6.2	2.0	0
peanuts, dry roasted	1 oz	160	14.1	6.7	6.1		0
peanuts, honey roasted	1 oz	150	13.0	6.0	5.0		0
peanuts, oil roasted	1 oz	165	14.0	7.5	5.4		0
peanuts, Spanish	1 oz	150	13.0	7.0	6.0	1.0	0
pecans, dry roasted	1 oz	187	18.3	2.3	6.3		0
pecans, oil roasted	1 oz	194	20.2	2.0	4.6		0
pine nuts	1 oz	160	14.4	6.8	4.0		0
pistachios, dry roasted	1 oz	172	15.0	4.2	7.8		0
sesame butter (tahini)	1 T	89	8.1	2.5	3.2		0
sunflower seeds, dry roasted	1 oz	165	14.1	5.5	6.8		0
sunflower seeds, oil roasted	1 oz	174	16.3	6.1	4.2		0
walnuts, dried	1 oz	190	19.0	4.0	4.0		0

OILS, SHORTENINGS, AND FATS

Food	Portion	Calories	Fat	Protein	Carb	Sugar	Chol
almond oil	1 T	124	14.0	0.0	0.0		0
avocado oil	1 T	124	14.0	0.0	0.0		0
Baker's Joy spray	1 spray	5	0.0	0.0	0.0		0
beef tallow	1 T	116	12.8	0.0	0.0		14
canola oil	1 T	124	14.0	0.0	0.0		0
chicken fat	1 T	117	13.0	0.0	0.0		11
corn oil	1 T	124	14.0	0.0	0.0		0
Crisco, butter flavor	1 T	110	12.0	0.0	0.0		0
Crisco oil	1 T	124	14.0	0.0	0.0		0
Crisco, regular	1 T	110	12.0	0.0	0.0		0

Food	Portion	Calories	Fat	Protein	Carb	Sugar	Chol
Harvest Blend, Fleischmann's	1 T	122	13.6	0.0	0.0		0
lard	1 T	117	13.0	0.0	0.0		12
Mazola No-Stick spray	1 spray	2	0.2	0.0	0.0		0
olive oil	1 T	124	14.0	0.0	0.0		0
peanut oil	1 T	124	14.0	0.0	0.0		0
Puritan vegetable oil	1 T	124	14.0	0.0	0.0		0
safflower oil	1 T	124	14.0	0.0	0.0		0
salt pork	1 oz	212	22.8	0.0	0.0		24
soybean oil	1 T	124	14.0	0.0	0.0		0
sunflower oil	1 T	124	14.0	0.0	0.0		0
vegetable oil, Wesson	1 T	124	14.0	0.0	0.0		0
walnut oil	1 T	124	14.0	0.0	0.0		0
wheat germ oil	1 T	124	14.0	0.0	0.0		0

PASTA, RICE, AND GRAINS

Food	Portion	Calories	Fat	Protein	Carb	Sugar	Chol
alfredo pasta primavera, Lean Cuisine	1 meal	280	6.0	12.0	44.0	5.0	10
angel hair pasta, Lean Cuisine	1 meal	240	4.0	9.0	43.0	11.0	5
angel hair pasta, Weight Watchers	1 meal	170	2.0	8.0	29.1		0
barley	¼ cup	166	1.1	5.2	36.7		0
bowtie pasta, marsala, Weight Watchers	1 meal	281	9.0	13.0	36.1		10
bowtie pasta, tomatoes, Lean Cuisine	1 meal	260	6.0	9.0	43.0		35
cavatelli, Celentano	1 cup	400	1.5	14.0	77.0	0.0	15
cheese cannelloni, Lean Cuisine	1 meal	250	6.0	16.0	30.0	9.0	20
egg noodles, cooked	1 cup	213	2.4	7.6	39.7		53

Food	Portion	Calories	Fat	Protein	Carb	Sugar	Chol
fettucini alfredo, Banquet	1 meal	370	18.0	12.0	39.0		30
fettucini alfredo, Lean Cuisine	1 meal	280	7.0	13.0	40.0	7.0	20
fettucini, chicken, Lean Cuisine	1 meal	270	6.0	21.0	33.0	5.0	40
fettucini, primavera, Budget Gourmet	1 meal	280	8.0	14.0	38.0		90
fettucini, turkey, Healthy Choice	1 meal	350	4.0	28.0	50.0		30
gnocchi, Celentano	1 cup	210	0.5	8.0	38.0	0.0	0
lasagna, cheese, Celentano	7 oz	270	12.0	11.0	29.0	4.0	50
lasagna, cheese, Lean Cuisine	1 meal	240	4.5	13.0	37.0	7.0	10
lasagna, chicken, Lean Cuisine	1 meal	280	7.0	20.0	34.0	6.0	40
lasagna, five cheese, Lean Cuisine	1 meal	210	5.0	14.0	27.0	6.0	20
lasagna, garden, Weight Watchers	1 meal	270	7.0	14.0	36.1		30
lasagna, meat, Budget Gourmet	1 meal	260	8.0	10.0	38.0		10
lasagna, meat sauce, Banquet	1 meal	290	9.0	14.0	39.0		10
lasagna, meat sauce, Lean Cuisine	1 meal	300	8.0	19.0	38.0	8.0	30
lasagna, meat sauce, Weight Watchers	1 meal	270	6.0	14.0	38.1		35
lasagna, vegetable, Banquet	1 meal	260	6.0	11.0	41.0		10
lasagna, vegetable, Celentano	10 oz	260	4.5	11.0	39.0	5.0	40

Food	Portion	Calories	Fat	Protein	Carb	Sugar	Chol
lasagna, vegetable, Lean Cuisine	1 meal	260	7.0	17.0	33.0	9.0	20
lasagna, zucchini, Healthy Choice	1 meal	330	1.5	20.0	58.0		10
lo mein, chicken, Banquet	1 meal	270	6.0	11.0	43.0		20
macaroni, cooked	1 cup	197	0.9	6.7	39.7		0
macaroni, beef, Banquet	1 cup	230	7.0	13.0	31.0		25
macaroni, beef, Healthy Choice	1 meal	211	2.2	14.0	33.0		14
macaroni, beef, Lean Cuisine	1 meal	260	5.0	16.0	38.0	8.0	25
macaroni, beef, Weight Watchers	1 meal	220	4.0	13.0	32.0		15
macaroni, cheese, Banquet	1 meal	350	12.0	13.0	47.0		20
macaroni, cheese, Lean Cuisine	1 meal	290	7.0	15.0	42.0	5.0	20
macaroni, cheese, Morton	1 meal	200	3.0	7.0	34.9		10
macaroni, cheese, Weight Watchers	1 meal	281	4.0	13.0	42.1		25
manicotti, cheese	1 meal	232	10.0	13.0	22.1		74
manicotti, cheese, Celentano	10 oz	340	16.0	13.0	34.0	6.0	60
manicotti, cheese, meat sauce	1 meal	243	11.0	15.1	20.1		86
manicotti, cheese, spinach, Lean Cuisine	1 meal	350	8.0	19.0	50.0	18.0	40
noodles, chicken, Banquet	1 cup	210	9.0	10.0	24.0		40
pasta, cheddar, broccoli, Banquet	1 meal	350	12.0	12.0	48.0		15
pasta, chicken, wine, Budget Gourmet	1 meal	270	7.0	13.0	39.0		25

Food	Portion	Calories	Fat	Protein	Carb	Sugar	Chol
pasta, Italian sausage, Banquet	1 meal	340	13.0	11.0	43.0		10
pasta, spinach Romano, Weight Watchers	1 meal	240	8.0	11.0	32.0		5
pasta, tomato basil, Weight Watchers	1 meal	260	9.0	12.0	33.0		10
penne pasta, ricotta, Weight Watchers	1 meal	280	6.0	12.0	45.0		5
penne pasta, tomato sauce, Lean Cuisine	1 meal	260	3.5	9.0	47.0	13.0	0
radiatore pasta, vegetables, Birdseye	1 cup	200	8.0	6.0	27.0	5.0	5
ravioli, cheese, Celetano	4 ravioli	260	6.0	12.0	40.0	2.0	45
ravioli, cheese, Healthy Choice	1 meal	250	4.0	11.0	44.0		20
ravioli, cheese, Lean Cuisine	1 meal	260	7.0	12.0	38.0	8.0	35
ravioli, cheese, Marie Callender's	1 cup	370	14.0	14.0	47.0		35
ravioli, cheese, Stouffer's	1 meal	380	13.0	15.0	51.0		100
ravioli, meat, Celentano	4 ravioli	270	5.0	11.0	44.0	1.0	35
rice, beans, Lean Cuisine	1 meal	300	5.0	10.0	54.0	10.0	15
rice, beans, Weight Watchers	1 meal	290	9.0	12.0	41.0		5
rice, broccoli, Green Giant	1 package	320	12.0	8.0	44.0		15
rice, brown, cooked	1 cup	216	1.8	5.0	44.8		0
rice, fried	1 cup	236	1.1	5.1	53.4	6.2	0
rice, fried, chicken, Chun King	1 meal	228	6.0	9.0	44.0		25

Food	Portion	Calories	Fat	Protein	Carb	Sugar	Chol
rice, fried, pork, Chun King	1 meal	290	6.0	11.0	48.0		25
rice, fried, vegetables, Budget Gourmet	1 meal	412	18.8	8.2	53.0		18
rice, Hunan-style, Weight Watchers	1 meal	250	7.0	7.0	39.1		5
rice, medley, Green Giant	1 package	240	3.0	6.0	46.0		5
rice, Mexican, Old El Paso	½ cup	110	2.0	8.0	90.0		0
rice, paella, Weight Watchers	1 meal	280	7.0	7.0	48.1		5
rice, pilaf Florentine, Weight Watchers	1 meal	290	7.0	9.0	47.0		5
rice, Spanish, Old El Paso	1 cup	130	1.0	3.0	28.0		0
rice, Spanish, Rice-a-Roni	2 oz	189	0.8	5.4	41.0	1.5	0
rice, white, cooked	1 cup	205	0.4	4.3	44.5		0
rice, yellow, Rice-a-Roni	2.5 oz	234	0.3	4.8	53.9	0.8	0
rigatoni, parmagiana, Marie Callender's	1 cup	300	14.0	12.0	32.0		25
roletti pasta, vegetables, Birdseye	1 cup	190	8.0	5.0	11.0	5.0	5
shells, stuffed, Celentano	10 oz	320	15.0	12.0	31.0	6.0	40
shells, stuffed, broccoli, Celentano	10 oz	230	4.5	10.0	32.0	5.0	20
soba noodles, cooked	1 cup	174	0.2	8.9	37.7		0
spaghetti, Bolognesa, Banquet	1 meal	370	16.0	14.0	40.0		35
spaghetti, cooked	1 cup	197	0.9	6.7	39.7		0

Food	Portion	Calories	Fat	Protein	Carb	Sugar	Chol
spaghetti, marinara, Budget Gourmet	1 meal	306	7.1	9.4	50.6		6
spaghetti, meatballs, Lean Cuisine	1 meal	270	6.0	18.0	37.0	6.0	20
spaghetti, meat sauce, Lean Cuisine	1 meal	300	5.0	13.0	51.0	9.0	15
spaghetti, meat sauce, Mortons	1 meal	170	3.0	6.0	30.0		5
spaghetti, meat sauce, Weight Watchers	1 meal	290	5.0	14.0	45.0		15
tortellini, meat	1 cup	340	4.0	21.0	55.0	4.0	35
tortellini, parmigiana, Birdseye	2¼ cups	240	12.0	9.0	25.0	5.0	25
tortellini, spinach-filled	1 cup	233	9.0	12.0	25.1		159
tuna noodle casserole, Weight Watchers	1 meal	270	4.0	13.0	39.0		35
wheat germ	¼ cup	111	3.1	8.4	14.4		0
wild rice, cooked	1 cup	166	0.6	6.5	35.0		0
ziti, baked, Celentano	9 oz	250	13.0	8.0	24.0	4.0	15

PIZZA

Food	Portion	Calories	Fat	Protein	Carb	Sugar	Chol
cheese, Amy's Kitchen	½ pizza	310	11.0	13.0	69.1		15
cheese, Jeno's	½ pizza	272	13.7	9.9	27.6		
cheese, John's	½ pizza	249	12.0	9.7	26.2		
cheese, Lean Cuisine	½ pizza	310	9.0	17.0	39.0		10
cheese, Stouffer's	½ pizza	300	5.0	15.0	49.0		10
cheese, microwave, Jeno's	1 pizza	242	11.0	10.0	25.0		15

Food	Portion	Calories	Fat	Protein	Carb	Sugar	Chol
cheese, microwave, Totino's	1 pizza	240	11.0	10.0	25.0		15
combination, Jeno's	½ pizza	520	28.0	17.0	49.0		25
combination, microwave, Totino's	1 pizza	310	18.0	11.0	25.0		15
creamy garlic, Lean Cuisine	½ pizza	310	7.0	15.0	47.0		15
deluxe combo, Weight Watchers	½ pizza	380	6.0	23.0	46.9		40
French bread, Healthy Choice	1 meal	310	4.0	20.0	49.0		10
French bread, cheese, Lean Cuisine	1 piece	300	5.0	15.0	49.0		10
French bread, pepperoni, Healthy Choice	1 meal	220	4.0	20.0	52.0		20
Hearty Pockets, chicken fajita	1 pocket	280	10.0	11.0	36.0		20
Hearty Pockets, pepperoni	1 pocket	350	17.0	15.0	35.0		30
Mexican style, microwave, Totino's	1 pizza	280	16.0	10.0	25.0		15
pepperoni, Jeno's	½ pizza	284	15.1	10.0	27.5		12
pepperoni, Lean Cuisine	½ pizza	340	12.0	18.0	40.0		25
pepperoni, Stouffer's	½ pizza	310	7.0	15.0	46.0		20
pepperoni, Weight Watchers	½ pizza	391	4.0	23.1	46.1		45
pizza bread, cheese, Stouffer's	1 piece	370	16.0	14.0	43.0		15
pizza bread, pepperoni, Stouffer's	1 piece	430	20.0	16.0	46.0		15

Food	Portion	Calories	Fat	Protein	Carb	Sugar	Chol
pizza bread, vegetable, Stouffer's	1 piece	380	16.0	14.0	46.0		20
sausage, microwave, Totino's	1 pizza	280	16.0	10.0	25.0		10
spinach, Amy's Kitchen	½ pizza	320	11.0	13.0	40.0		15
sun-dried tomato, Lean Cuisine	½ pizza	340	8.0	19.0	48.0		20

POULTRY AND EGGS
EGGS

Food	Portion	Calories	Fat	Protein	Carb	Sugar	Chol
egg, hard/soft boiled	1 large egg	78	5.3	6.3	0.6		212
egg, fried	1 large egg	92	6.9	6.2	0.6		211
egg, poached	1 large egg	75	5.0	6.2	0.6		212
egg, scrambled	1 large egg	93	7.0	6.3	0.6		214
egg, white only	1 large egg	17	0.0	3.5	0.3		0
egg, yolk only	1 large egg	61	5.2	2.8	0.3		218

CHICKEN

Food	Portion	Calories	Fat	Protein	Carb	Sugar	Chol
breast, fried, no skin	½ breast	161	4.1	28.8	0.4		78
breast, roasted, no skin	½ breast	142	3.1	26.7	0.0		73
breast, fried, with skin	½ breast	218	8.7	31.2	1.6		87
breast, roasted, with skin	½ breast	193	7.6	29.2	0.0		82
drumstick, roasted, no skin	1 drumstick	76	2.5	12.4	0.0		41
drumstick, fried, with skin	1 drumstick	120	6.7	13.2	0.8		44
drumstick, roasted, with skin	1 drumstick	112	5.8	14.1	0.0		47
liver, braised	3.5 oz	157	5.5	24.4	0.9		631
thigh, roasted, no skin	1 thigh	109	5.7	13.5	0.0		49

Food	Portion	Calories	Fat	Protein	Carb	Sugar	Chol
thigh, fried, with skin	1 thigh	162	9.3	16.6	2.0		60
thigh, roasted, with skin	1 thigh	153	9.6	15.5	0.0		58
wing, fried, with skin	1 wing	103	7.1	8.4	0.8		26
wing, roasted, with skin	1 wing	99	6.6	9.1	0.0		29
DUCK							
duck, roasted, no skin	3.5 oz	201	11.2	23.5	0.0		89
duck, roasted, with skin	3.5 oz	337	28.4	19.0	0.0		84
TURKEY							
bacon	1 slice	34	2.7	2.2	0.2	0.2	13
breast, roasted, no skin	3.5 oz	157	3.2	29.9	0.0		69
breast, roasted, with skin	3.5 oz	197	8.3	28.6	0.0		76
dark meat, roasted, no skin	3.5 oz	187	7.2	28.6	0.0		85
dark meat, roasted, with skin	3.5 oz	221	11.5	27.5	0.0		89
ground	3.5 oz	170	9.8	20.6	0.0		84
SNACK FOODS							
Bugles	1⅓ cups	150	7.0	1.0	20.0	1.0	0
Bugles, baked	1½ cups	130	3.5	2.0	23.0	2.0	0
Bugles, nacho	1⅓ cups	160	9.0	2.0	18.0	2.0	0
Bugles, ranch	1⅓ cups	160	9.0	2.0	18.0	2.0	0
Bugles, sour cream and onion	1⅓ cups	160	9.0	2.0	20.0	2.0	0
cheese puffs/twists	1 oz	157	9.8	2.2	15.3		1
Cheetos, curls	15 chips	150	10.0	2.0	15.0		0
Cheetos, nacho cheese	23 chips	160	10.0	2.0	15.0		0

Food	Portion	Calories	Fat	Protein	Carb	Sugar	Chol
Cheetos, puffed balls	38 chips	150	10.0	2.0	15.0		0
Cheetos, puffs	29 chips	160	10.0	2.0	15.0		0
Cheez Curls, Planters	1 oz	150	10.0	2.0	15.0	1.0	
Cheez Curls, reduced fat, Planters	1 oz	130	5.0	3.0	19.0	1.0	
Chex Mix	2 oz	242	9.9	6.0	37.2		0
Combos Pretzel Cheddar Snacks	10 combos	139	5.1	3.0	20.0		2
corn cakes	2 cakes	70	0.4	1.5	15.0		0
corn cakes, caramel, Quaker	1 cake	50	0.2	0.7	11.5	3.8	0
corn cakes, blueberry crunch, Quaker	1 cake	49	0.2	0.7	11.5	3.9	0
corn cakes, butter flavor, Quaker	1 cake	34	0.2	0.7	7.5	0.0	0
corn cakes, white cheddar, Quaker	1 cake	38	0.3	0.9	8.1	0.4	0
corn chips	1 oz	153	9.5	1.9	16.1		0
corn chips, barbecue	1 oz	148	9.3	2.0	15.9		0
Cracker Jack	½ cup	120	2.0	2.0	23.0	15.0	0
Doritos, corn	12 chips	140	7.0	2.0	18.0	1.0	0
Doritos, Flamin' Hot	11 chips	140	7.0	2.0	17.0		0
Doritos, nacho cheese	12 chips	140	7.0	2.0	18.0	1.0	0
Doritos, ranch	12 chips	140	7.0	2.0	18.0		0
Doritos, spicy nacho	12 chips	140	6.0	2.0	18.0		0
Fritos	29 chips	160	10.0	2.0	15.0	1.0	0
Fritos, BBQ	29 chips	150	9.0	2.0	16.0		0
Fritos, chili cheese	31 chips	160	10.0	2.0	16.0		0
Funyuns, Frito-Lay	13 chips	140	7.0	2.0	18.0		0
popcorn, caramel	1 cup	151	4.5	1.3	27.7	13.8	2

Food	Portion	Calories	Fat	Protein	Carb	Sugar	Chol
popcorn, caramel, Fiddle Faddle	¾ cup	150	7.0	2.0	20.0	12.0	10
popcorn, cheese, Pop Secret	1 cup	30	2.0	2.6	14.4		0
popcorn, cheese, Redenbacher	2 T unpopped	169	13.0	1.0	23.0	12.0	0
popcorn, Pop Secret	1 cup	35	2.5	4.0	0.0		0
popcorn, Redenbacher	2 T unpopped	168	12.5	3.0	22.0	0.0	0
popcorn cakes	2 cakes	77	0.6	1.9	16.0		0
popcorn cakes, caramel, Quaker	1 cake	47	0.3	1.0	11.2	3.8	0
potato chips, baked, Lay's	11 chips	110	1.5	2.0	23.0		0
potato chips, BBQ flavor	1 oz	148	9.3	2.0	15.8		0
potato chips, BBQ, Lay's	15 chips	150	10.0	2.0	15.0		0
potato chips, deli style, Lay's	17 chips	150	10.0	2.0	16.0		0
potato chips, Flamin' Hot, Lay's	17 chips	150	10.0	2.0	16.0		0
potato chips, onion, garlic, Lay's	19 chips	150	9.0	2.0	16.0		0
potato chips, onion, garlic, Utz	1 oz	150	9.0	2.1	14.6		0
potato chips, plain	1 oz	152	9.8	2.0	15.0		0
potato chips, salt, vinegar, Lay's	17 chips	150	10.0	2.0	15.0		0
potato chips, sour cream, onion	1 oz	151	9.6	2.3	14.6		2
potato chips, sour cream, onion, Lay's	12 chips	160	11.0	2.0	12.0		0
potato chips, Utz	1 oz	150	9.0	2.0	14.9		0
pretzels, cheddar, Rold Gold	17 pretzels	110	0.0	3.0	23.0		0

Food	Portion	Calories	Fat	Protein	Carb	Sugar	Chol
pretzels, chocolate-coated	1 oz	128	4.7	2.1	19.9		0
pretzels, Dutch, Mr. Salty	2 pretzels	120	1.0	3.0	25.0		0
pretzels, honey mustard	17 pretzels	110	0.0	3.0	23.0		0
pretzels, honey mustard, onion, Snyder's	13 pretzels	130	3.0	3.0	23.0		0
pretzels, sourdough, Snyder's	16 pretzels	120	0.0	3.0	25.0		0
pretzels, sourdough nuggets	11 pretzels	110	0.0	2.0	24.0		0
pretzels, sticks, Rold Gold	48 pretzels	110	0.0	3.0	23.0		0
pretzels, thin, Rold Gold	4 pretzels	110	1.5	3.0	22.0		0
pretzels, tiny twists, Rold Gold	18 pretzels	100	0.0	3.0	23.0		0
pretzels, twists, Mr. Salty	9 pretzels	110	0.0	3.0	23.0		0
Pringle's potato crips	1 oz	160	11.0	2.0	15.0		0
rice cakes, Quaker	1 cake	35	0.3	0.8	7.5		0
rice cakes, banana nut, Quaker	1 cake	50	0.3	0.7	11.4	5.0	0
rice cakes, chocolate crunch, Quaker	1 cake	50	0.3	0.9	11.2	3.8	0
Ruffles, baked	10 chips	110	1.5	2.0	23.0		0
Ruffles, baked, sour cream, onions	9 chips	120	3.0	2.0	21.0		0
Ruffles, cheddar, sour cream	11 chips	160	10.0	2.0	14.0		0
Ruffles, French onion	11 chips	150	10.0	2.0	15.0		0

Food	Portion	Calories	Fat	Protein	Carb	Sugar	Chol
Ruffles, original	12 chips	160	10.0	2.0	14.0		0
Ruffles, ranch	13 chips	150	9.0	2.0	15.0		0
Ruffles, reduced fat	16 chips	130	6.7	2.0	18.0		0
Sun Chips	14 chips	140	6.0	2.0	19.0		0
Sun Chips, French onion	13 chips	140	7.0	2.0	18.0		0
Sun Chips, harvest cheddar	13 chips	140	6.0	2.0	19.0		0
tortilla chips	1 oz	142	7.4	2.0	17.8		0
tortilla chips, baked	1 oz	120	1.5	2.0	16.4		0
tortilla chips, nacho	1 oz	141	7.3	2.2	17.7		1
tortilla chips, ranch	1 oz	139	6.7	2.2	18.3		0
tortilla chips, taco flavor	1 oz	136	6.9	2.2	17.9		1
Tostitos, baked	13 chips	110	1.0	3.0	21.0		0
Tostitos, lime, chili	6 chips	150	7.0	2.0	17.0		0
Tostitos, nacho	6 chips	150	6.0	2.0	19.0		0
Tostitos, restaurant-style	7 chips	140	6.0	2.0	19.0		0
Tostitos, salsa, cheese	6 chips	140	7.0	2.0	18.0		0
Tostitos, salsa, cream cheese	16 chips	120	3.0	2.0	21.0		3
SOUP, PREPARED							
bean with bacon	½ cup	180	5.0	8.0	25.0	4.0	3
beef broth	½ cup	15	0.0	3.0	1.0		3
beef, chunky	½ cup	85	2.5	5.0	11.0	1.0	7
beef mushroom	½ cup	32	1.5	5.0	6.0	1.0	4
beef noodle	½ cup	70	2.5	5.0	8.0	1.0	15
black bean	½ cup	120	2.0	6.0	19.0	4.0	0
broccoli cheese	½ cup	110	7.0	3.0	9.0	2.0	10
broccoli, cream of	½ cup	100	6.0	3.3	14.9	0.5	3
celery, cream of	½ cup	82	4.6	4.0	21.4		16

Food	Portion	Calories	Fat	Protein	Carb	Sugar	Chol
cheese, cheddar	½ cup	90	4.0	4.0	10.0	2.0	15
chicken alphabet	½ cup	80	2.0	4.0	11.0	1.0	10
chicken broth	½ cup	30	2.0	2.0	2.0	1.0	3
chicken, chunky	½ cup	84	3.3	6.2	8.1		15
chicken, creamy	½ cup	130	7.0	5.0	12.0	2.0	15
chicken noodle	½ cup	70	2.0	3.0	9.0	1.0	15
chicken rice	½ cup	70	2.5	3.0	9.0	0.0	3
clam chowder, Manhattan	½ cup	60	0.5	2.0	12.0	2.0	3
clam chowder, New England	½ cup	100	2.5	4.0	15.0	1.0	3
lentil	½ cup	65	0.4	4.4	13.6	1.0	0
lentil, ham	½ cup	70	1.4	4.1	10.1		4
minestrone	½ cup	100	2.0	5.0	16.0	3.0	0
mushroom barley	½ cup	36	1.1	1.0	6.0		0
mushroom, cream of	½ cup	110	7.0	2.0	9.0	1.0	3
onion	½ cup	29	0.9	2.0	7.6		0
pea, split, with ham	½ cup	180	3.5	10.0	28.0	4.0	3
pepperpot	½ cup	100	5.0	4.0	9.0	1.0	15
ramen noodle	1 package	290	11.0	6.0	41.0	3.0	0
tomato	½ cup	100	2.0	5.0	40.3		0
tomato bisque	½ cup	130	3.0	2.0	24.0	15.0	5
tomato rice	½ cup	120	2.0	23.0	11.0		5
turkey, chunky	½ cup	70	2.2	5.1	7.1		5
turkey noodle	½ cup	80	2.5	4.0	10.0	1.0	15
vegetable, beef	½ cup	80	2.0	5.0	10.0	2.0	10
vegetable, chunky	½ cup	61	1.4	1.4	9.0		0
vegetarian	½ cup	70	1.0	2.0	14.0	6.0	0

SUGAR AND OTHER SWEETENERS

corn syrup, dark	1 T	56	0.0	0.0	15.3	7.4	0
corn syrup, light	1 T	56	0.0	0.0	15.3	12.7	0
maple syrup	1 T	52	0.0	0.0	13.4	12.0	0
molasses	1 T	53	0.0	0.0	13.8	10.9	0

Calorie Counts for Common Food...

Food	Portion	Calories	Fat	Protein	Carb		
molasses, blackstrap	1 T	47	0.0	0.0	12.2	9.0	
pancake syrup, Aunt Jemima	¼ cup	212	0.0	0.0	52.6	37.8	0
pancake syrup, Aunt Jemima butter lite	¼ cup	104	0.0	0.0	26.4	26.0	0
pancake syrup, Aunt Jemima butter rich	¼ cup	209	0.2	0.1	51.9	28.9	0
pancake syrup, Log Cabin	¼ cup	200	0.0	0.0	52.0	31.0	0
pancake syrup, Log Cabin lite	¼ cup	100	0.0	0.0	26.0	25.0	0
pancake syrup, Mrs. Butterworth	1 T	55	0.0	0.0	27.0		0
pancake syrup, Mrs. Butterworth lite	1 T	31	0.1	0.0	8.0		0
sugar, brown	1 cup	827	0.0	0.0	214.0	197.5	0
sugar, turbinado	1 t	15	0.0	0.0	4.0	3.9	0
sugar, white granulated	1 t	15	0.0	0.0	4.0	3.9	0
sugar, white granulated	1 T	50	0.0	0.0	13.0	12.6	0
sugar, white granulated	1 cup	774	0.0	0.0	199.8	193.6	0
sugar, white, confectioner's	1 T	31	0.0	0.0	8.0	7.4	0
VEGETABLES							
alfalfa sprouts, raw	1 cup	10	0.0	1.3	1.2		0
arugula, raw	½ cup	3	0.0	0.3	0.4		0
asparagus, boiled	½ cup	22	0.3	2.3	3.8	1.4	0
bamboo shoots, canned	1 cup	25	0.5	2.3	4.2		0
Bavarian-style, Birdseye	½ cup	150	8.0	5.0	15.0	3.0	30

Food	Portion	Calories	Fat	Protein	Carb	Sugar	Chol
bean sprouts, canned	1 cup	11	0.1	1.3	1.2		0
beans, baked, Campbell's	½ cup	180	3.0	5.0	32.0	14.0	5
beans, chili	½ cup	130	3.0	6.0	21.0	4.0	5
beans, chili, Stouffer's	1 cup	270	10.0	15.0	29.0		35
beans, Mexe, Old El Paso	½ cup	110	0.5	7.0	19.0		0
beans, refried, Old El Paso	½ cup	110	2.0	6.0	17.0		5
beans, refried, cheese, Old El Paso	½ cup	130	3.5	7.0	18.0		5
beans with pork, Campbell's	½ cup	130	2.0	5.0	24.0	8.0	5
beans with pork, Hunt's	½ cup	130	1.2	6.2	27.5	16.4	0
beets, canned	½ cup	26	0.1	0.8	6.1		0
black beans, cooked	1 cup	227	0.9	15.2	40.8		0
black-eyed peas, canned	½ cup	91	0.6	7.1	17.8		0
broccoli, au gratin, Stouffer's	½ cup	100	4.0	5.0	10.0		10
broccoli, cauliflower, carrots, cheese	½ cup	70	4.0	3.0	7.0	3.0	5
broccoli, frozen	½ cup	26	0.1	2.9	4.9		0
broccoli, frozen, butter sauce	½ cup	40	2.0	2.1	5.9		5
broccoli, frozen, cheese sauce	½ cup	116	6.2	4.8	11.6		6
Brussels sprouts, frozen	½ cup	33	0.3	2.8	6.5		0
Brussels sprouts, frozen, butter sauce	½ cup	40	1.0	2.9	8.0		5
Brussels sprouts, frozen, cheese sauce	½ cup	113	5.6	5.0	12.5		5

Food	Portion	Calories	Fat	Protein	Carb	Sugar	Chol
butter beans, canned	½ cup	76	0.4	5.7	15.9		0
cabbage, green, raw	½ cup	9	0.1	0.5	1.9	1.3	0
California-style, Birdseye	½ cup	100	5.0	3.0	9.0	4.0	10
carrots, boiled	½ cup	35	0.1	0.9	8.2	3.4	0
carrots, raw	1 medium	31	0.1	0.7	7.3	4.8	0
cauliflower, frozen	½ cup	17	0.2	1.4	3.4		0
cauliflower, frozen, butter sauce	½ cup	30	1.2	1.1	3.5		
cauliflower, frozen, cheese sauce	½ cup	114	6.1	4.0	11.7		6
celery, raw	1 stalk	6	0.1	0.3	1.5	0.4	0
chard, Swiss, cooked	½ cup	18	0.1	1.7	3.6		0
chickpeas, canned	1 cup	286	2.7	11.9	54.3		0
chickpea hummus	½ cup	210	10.4				0
chicory, raw	½ cup	21	0.3	1.5	4.2		0
chili, beans, Old El Paso	1 cup	200	7.0	19.0	15.0		30
chili, black beans, Health Valley	½ cup	70	0.0	7.0	9.0		0
Chinese-style, Birdseye	½ cup	68	3.9	2.2	7.7		0
coleslaw	½ cup	41	1.6	0.8	7.4		5
collards, boiled	½ cup	31	0.3	2.5	6.0		0
corn, kernels, canned	½ cup	66	0.8	2.1	15.2	2.3	0
corn, cream style, canned	½ cup	59	0.3	1.4	14.9		0
corn, gold and white, Birdseye	½ cup	60	1.0	2.0	11.0	4.0	0
corn, souffle, Stouffer's	½ cup	170	7.0	5.0	21.0		65
cranberry beans, canned	½ cup	108	0.5	7.2	20.0		0

Food	Portion	Calories	Fat	Protein	Carb	Sugar	Chol
cucumber, raw	½ cup	7	0.1	0.4	1.4		0
dandelion greens, raw	½ cup	13	0.2	0.8	2.6		0
eggplant, boiled	½ cup	13	0.1	0.4	3.2		0
eggplant, fried sticks	½ cup	240	12.3	4.1	28.2		
eggplant, parmagiana, frozen	½ cup	264	16.4	6.4	25.8		7
endive, raw	½ cup	4	0.1	0.3	0.8		0
French-style, Birdseye	⅔ cup	110	6.0	2.0	10.0	2.0	10
garlic, raw	3 cloves	13	0.0	0.6	3.0		0
great northern beans, canned	½ cup	150	0.5	9.1	24.6		0
green beans, frozen	½ cup	19	0.1	1.0	4.4		0
green beans, almonds, frozen	½ cup	52	1.6	2.5	8.4		0
green beans, butter sauce, frozen	½ cup	52	2.8	1.7	8.4		5
green beans casserole, Stouffer's	½ cup	140	2.0	3.0	13.0		10
hominy, white, canned	1 cup	115	1.4	2.4	22.8		0
Italian-style, Birdseye	½ cup	102	5.5	2.1	11.1		0
Japanese-style, Birdseye	½ cup	89	5.0	2.0	10.0		0
kale, cooked	½ cup	21	0.3	1.2	3.7		0
kidney beans, canned	1 cup	207	0.8	13.3	38.1		0
leeks, cooked	½ cup	16	0.2	0.4	4.0		0
lentils, cooked	1 cup	230	0.8	17.9	39.9		0
lettuce, iceberg	1 leaf	2	0.0	0.2	0.4		0
lettuce, romaine, raw	½ cup	4	0.1	0.5	0.7		0

Food	Portion	Calories	Fat	Protein	Carb	Sugar	Chol
lima beans, frozen	½ cup	85	0.3	5.2	16.0		0
lima beans, butter sauce, frozen	½ cup	100	3.0	6.0	17.0		5
onions, cream sauce, frozen	½ cup	100	5.9				
Mexican-style, Birdseye	½ cup	141	4.9	4.9	23.5		
mixed vegetables, frozen	½ cup	54	0.1	2.6	11.9		0
mushrooms, raw	½ cup	9	0.1	0.7	1.6		0
mustard greens, cooked	½ cup	14	0.2	1.7	2.3		0
navy beans, canned	1 cup	296	1.1	19.7	53.6		0
New England-style, pasta, Birdseye	1 cup	260	14.0	6.0	29.0	6.0	15
okra, cooked	½ cup	30	0.2	1.7	4.6		0
okra, breaded	½ cup	166	9.6	3.0	17.0		4
onion rings, frozen	7 rings	285	18.7	3.7	26.7		0
onions, raw	½ cup	30	0.1	0.9	6.9		0
Oriental, lo mein, Birdseye	2¼ cups	230	3.5	8.0	40.0	11.0	5
Oriental-style, Birdseye	½ cup	60	4.0	2.0	4.0	3.0	0
parsnips, boiled	½ cup	63	0.2	1.0	15.2		0
pearl onions, cream sauce	½ cup	60	2.0	2.0	8.0	6.0	10
peas and carrots, frozen	½ cup	38	0.3	2.5	8.1		0
peas and pearl onions, frozen	½ cup	71	0.2	4.6	13.5		0
peas, frozen	½ cup	62	0.2	4.1	11.4		0
peas, cream sauce, frozen	½ cup	118	5.6	4.1	13.4		1
peas, split, cooked	1 cup	231	0.8	16.3	41.4		0
peppers, stuffed, Stouffer's	1 cup	200	5.0	11.0	27.0		20

Food	Portion	Calories	Fat	Protein	Carb	Sugar	Chol
peppers, sweet, raw	½ cup	14	0.1	0.4	3.2		0
pink beans, canned	1 cup	252	0.8	15.3	47.2		0
pinto beans, canned	1 cup	206	1.9	11.7	36.6		0
potato, baked with skin	1 potato	220	0.2	4.6	51.0		0
potato, baked, broccoli, cheese	1 potato	250	7.0	12.0	35.0		10
potato, cheddar cheese, frozen	1 potato	228	10.8	6.3	27.5		6
potato puffs, frozen	½ cup	138	6.7	2.1	18.9		0
potato salad	½ cup	179	10.3	3.4	14.0		85
potatoes, au gratin, frozen	½ cup	161	9.3	6.0	17.9		28
potatoes, au gratin, mix	½ cup	127	5.6	3.2	17.6		21
potatoes, au gratin, Stouffer's	½ cup	130	6.0	4.0	15.0		15
potatoes, cottage fries, frozen	½ cup	109	4.1	2.2	19.5		0
potatoes, french fries, frozen	½ cup	167	9.4	2.2	23.7		0
potatoes, hash brown, frozen	½ cup	163	10.8	1.9	16.6		0
potatoes, mashed, flakes	½ cup	119	5.9	2.0	15.8		15
potatoes, roasted, broccoli, Birdseye	⅔ cup	100	3.5	3.0	15.0	2.0	0
potatoes, scalloped, frozen	½ cup	98	3.5	3.7	12.7		8
potatoes, scalloped, mix	½ cup	127	5.9	2.9	17.5		15
potatoes, scalloped, Stouffer's	½ cup	140	5.0	4.0	19.0		3
potatoes, Tater Tots, frozen	½ cup	161	7.3	2.4	21.3		0

Food	Portion	Calories	Fat	Protein	Carb	Sugar	Chol
pumpkin, canned	½ cup	41	0.3	1.3	9.9		0
radicchio, raw	½ cup	5	0.1	0.3	0.9		0
radish, raw	10 radishes	8	0.2	0.3	1.6		0
red beans, canned	½ cup	89	0.5	6.2	18.9		0
rhubarb, frozen, cooked	½ cup	139	0.1	0.5	37.4		0
rice, broccoli, cheese sauce, Birdseye	1 package	290	9.0	8.0	15.0	4.0	15
rice, wild rice, green beans, Birdseye	1 cup	180	4.0	4.0	31.0	2.0	10
snow peas, frozen	½ cup	40	1.5	2.3	4.4		0
spinach, boiled	½ cup	21	0.2	2.7	3.4		0
spinach, butter sauce, frozen	½ cup	40	2.0	3.0	6.0		5
spinach, creamed, frozen	½ cup	60	2.0	2.1	5.1		2
spinach, souffle, Stouffer's	½ cup	150	10.0	6.0	9.0		120
squash, acorn, baked	½ cup	57	0.1	1.1	14.9		0
squash, butternut, baked	½ cup	41	0.1	0.9	10.7		0
squash, summer, cooked	½ cup	18	0.3	0.8	3.9		0
stir-fry style, Birdseye	½ cup	60	4.0	2.0	5.0	4.0	10
succotash, frozen	½ cup	79	0.8	3.7	17.0		0
sweet potato, baked	1 sweet potato	117	0.1	2.0	27.7		0
sweet potato, mashed	½ cup	172	0.5	1.0	24.9		0
sweet potato, syrup, canned	½ cup	106	0.3	1.3	24.9		0
sweet potato, whipped, frozen	½ cup	139	5.5	2.1	17.5		16
tomato paste	2 T	30	0.5	1.0	5.7	3.7	0
tomato puree, canned	1 cup	100	0.4	4.2	23.9		0

Food	Portion	Calories	Fat	Protein	Carb	Sugar	Chol
tomato, raw	1 tomato	26	0.4	1.0	5.7		0
turnip, cooked	½ cup	14	0.1	0.6	3.8		0
turnip greens, cooked	½ cup	14	0.2	0.8	3.1		0
water chestnuts, canned	½ cup	35	0.0	0.6	8.7		0
watercress, raw	½ cup	2	0.0	0.4	0.2		0
wax beans, canned	½ cup	25	0.2	1.3	4.5		0
white beans, canned	1 cup	307	0.8	19.0	57.5		0
zucchini, cooked	½ cup	14	0.0	0.6	3.5		0
zucchini, breaded, frozen	½ cup	168	10.0	3.7	15.9		3

INDEX